The Anthropology of Epidemics

Over the past decades, infectious disease epidemics have come to increasingly pose major global health challenges to humanity. *The Anthropology of Epidemics* approaches epidemics as total social phenomena: processes and events which encompass and exercise a transformational impact on social life whilst at the same time functioning as catalysts of shifts and ruptures as regards human/non-human relations. Bearing a particular mark on subject areas and questions which have recently come to shape developments in anthropological thinking, the volume brings epidemics to the forefront of anthropological debate, as an exemplary arena for social scientific study and analysis.

Ann H. Kelly is Senior Lecturer in the Department of Global Health and Social Medicine, King's College London, UK, and Co-Deputy Director of the King's Global Health Institute. Her work focuses on the socio-material practices of global health research and innovation in sub-Saharan Africa.

Frédéric Keck is Director of Research at CNRS, attached to the Laboratory for Social Anthropology in Paris, France. He has conducted researches on the genealogy of social sciences, the ethnography of zoonotic diseases, and the microbial history of collections of human remains.

Christos Lynteris is Senior Lecturer in Social Anthropology at the University of St Andrews, UK. His work focuses on the anthropological and historical examination of infectious disease epidemics. He is the author of *The Spirit of Selflessness in Maoist China* (2012) and *Ethnographic Plague* (2016).

Routledge Studies in Health and Medical Anthropology

Depression in Kerala
Ayurveda and Mental Health Care in 21st Century India
Claudia Lang

Diagnosis Narratives and the Healing Ritual in Western Medicine
James P. Meza

The Anthropology of Epidemics
Edited by Ann H. Kelly, Frédéric Keck and Christos Lynteris

Haemophilia in Aotearoa New Zealand
Julie Park, Kathryn M. Scott, Deon York, and Michael Carnahan

www.routledge.com/Routledge-Studies-in-Health-and-Medical-Anthropology/book-series/RSHMA

The Anthropology of Epidemics

Edited by Ann H. Kelly, Frédéric Keck
and Christos Lynteris

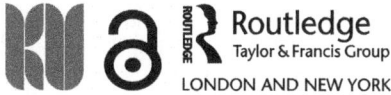

Routledge
Taylor & Francis Group
LONDON AND NEW YORK

First published 2019
by Routledge
2 Park Square, Milton Park, Abingdon, Oxon OX14 4RN

and by Routledge
52 Vanderbilt Avenue, New York, NY 10017

First issued in paperback 2020

Routledge is an imprint of the Taylor & Francis Group, an informa business

British Library Cataloguing-in-Publication Data
A catalogue record for this book is available from the British Library

Library of Congress Cataloging-in-Publication Data
A catalog record for this book has been requested

ISBN 13: 978-0-367-58194-7 (pbk)
ISBN 13: 978-1-138-61667-7 (hbk)

DOI: 10.4324/9780429461897

Contents

Figures

Contributors

Hannah Brown is Lecturer in the Department of Anthropology at Durham University, UK. Her research centres on the topics of work, health and development, and on the ways people care for one another through institutional and interpersonal mechanisms. She has worked in Kenya and Sierra Leone. Recent publications include a volume co-edited with Ruth Prince, *Volunteer Economies: The Politics and Ethics of Voluntary Labour in Africa* (James Currey, 2016); a special issue of the *Journal of the Royal Anthropological Institute*, 'Meetings: Ethnographies of Organisational, Process, Bureaucracy and Assembly'; and a special issue of *Medical Anthropology Quarterly*, 'Humans, Animals and Health' (co-edited with Alex Nading). Her current research explores the field of human-animal health and epidemic management in development contexts.

Carlo Caduff is Senior Lecturer in the Department of Global Health and Social Medicine at King's College London, UK. He received his PhD in Anthropology from the University of California at Berkeley, USA. His research explores the politics of bioscience, biomedicine, and biosecurity in the United States and India. His first book – *The Pandemic Perhaps* – was published by the University of California Press in 2015. He serves as Director of Postgraduate Research Studies and Chair of the Culture, Medicine & Power Research Group (CMP) in the Department of Global Health and Social Medicine. He is Associate Faculty at the India Institute and Visiting Faculty at the Graduate Institute Geneva.

Frédéric Keck is Director of Research at CNRS, Paris, France, based at the Laboratory for Social Anthropology. He has worked on the history of social anthropology and the contemporary management of zoonotic diseases. He has coordinated the research project 'Social Représentations of Pathogens at the Border Between Species' supported by the Axa Research Fund at the Collège de France, and directed the Department of Research and Education at the Musée du quai Branly in Paris. He published *Claude Lévi-Strauss, une introduction* (Pocket-La découverte, 2005), *Lucien Lévy-Bruhl, entre philosophie et anthropologie* (CNRS Editions, 2008), and *Un monde grippé* (Flammarion, 2010). He has co-edited as special issues (with Noelie Vialles) *Des hommes malades des animaux*, L'Herne, 2012 (with Andrew Lakoff) 'Sentinel devices', *Limn*,

2013, and (with Christos Lynteris) 'Zoonosis', *Medicine Anthropology Theory*, 2018. He will soon publish *Avian Reservoirs: Virus Hunters and Birdwatchers in Chinese Sentinel Posts* (Duke University Press).

Ann H. Kelly is Senior Lecturer in the Department of Global Health and Social Medicine, King's College London, UK, and the Co-Deputy Director of the King's Global Health Institute. Her ethnographic work focuses on the socio-material practices of global health research and innovation in sub-Saharan Africa, recent examples of which have been published in *Cultural Anthropology*, *Social Studies of Science*, *Social Science and Medicine* and *Visual Anthropology*. She is currently collaborating on a number of transdisciplinary initiatives including an NIHR Research Unit on System Strengthening in sub-Saharan Africa (ASSET) and, with colleagues at the University of Edinburgh and the Indian Institute of Public Health–Hyderabad, an ERC-funded project investigating the Design and Use of Diagnostic Devices in Global Health (Dia-Dev). She currently serves as a member of the Working Group on Ebola Vaccines of the WHO's Strategic Advisory Group of Experts (SAGE).

Guillaume Lachenal is Associate Professor in History of Science at the Université Paris Diderot, France. He studies the history and anthropology of biomedicine in Africa. He has coordinated the Agence Nationale de la Recherche (ANR) project 'Memorials and remains of medical research in Africa' (MEREAF), an anthropological and archaeological exploration of the ruins and memories associated with the past in African medical institutions. He has published *Le médicament qui devait sauver l'Afrique. Un scandale pharmaceutique aux colonies* (La Découverte, 2014), and *Le médecin qui voulut être roi. Sur les traces d'une utopie coloniale* (Le Seuil, 2017). He has co-edited *Politiques de la nostalgie* for *Politique Africaine* (2014), with Aïssatou Mbodj-Pouye, *La médecine du tri. Histoire, anthropologie, éthique* (Presses Universitaires de France, 2014), with Céline Lefève and Vinh-Kim Nguyen, and *Traces of the Future: An Archaeology of Medical Science in Africa* (Intellect, 2016), with Wenzel Geissler, John Manton, and Noemi Tousignant.

Andrew Lakoff is Professor of Sociology and Communication at the University of Southern California, USA. He is the author of *Pharmaceutical Reason: Knowledge and Value in Global Psychiatry* (Cambridge, 2006) and *Unprepared: Global Health in a Time of Emergency* (University of California, 2017), and is co-editor (with Stephen J. Collier) of *Biosecurity Interventions: Global Health and Security in Question* (Columbia, 2008).

Christos Lynteris is Senior Lecturer in Social Anthropology at the University of St Andrews, UK. A medical anthropologist investigating epistemological, biopolitical, and aesthetic aspects of infectious disease epidemics, he was the recipient of an ERC Starting Grant for the project 'Visual Representations of the Third Plague Pandemic' (University of Cambridge/University of St Andrews, 2013–18). He is the author of *The Spirit of Selflessness in Maoist China: Socialist Medicine and the New Man* (Palgrave, 2012) and *Ethnographic Plague:*

Configuring Disease on the Chinese-Russian Frontier (Palgrave, 2016). He has co-edited *Histories of Post-Mortem Contagion: Infectious Corpses and Contested Burials* (Palgrave, 2018) with Nicholas Evans, *Plague and the City* (Routledge, 2018) with Lukas Engelmann and John Henderson, and several special issues, including, most recently, 'Zoonosis', for *Medicine Anthropology Theory* (2018) with Frédéric Keck, and 'Technologies and Materialities of Epidemic Control', for *Medical Anthropology* (2018) with Branwyn Poleykett.

Vinh-Kim Nguyen is a medical anthropologist and physician. As a clinician he has specialised in HIV care, working in dedicated clinics in Canada and West Africa, while continuing general acute care practice as an emergency physician and hospitalist at the Jewish General Hospital in Montreal, Canada. He has also practiced emergency medicine at the Hôpital Avicenne in Paris, and with Médecins sans Frontières in conflict zones in the Middle East. He was part of the front-line response to the Ebola epidemic in 2014, where he coordinated a team of anthropologists assisting efforts to develop effective treatments and vaccines. His current research focuses on efforts to eliminate HIV transmission through novel biomedical and social technologies, and the linkages between conflict, environmental degradation, and antimicrobial resistance. He teaches at the Graduate Institute in Geneva, holds appointments in the Schools of Public Health in Beirut and Montreal, and currently advises Inserm, MSF, and the WHO on global health issues. His first book, *The Republic of Therapy: Triage and Sovereignty in West Africa's Time of AIDS*, is currently in its second printing. With Margaret Lock, he is the co-author of *An Anthropology of Biomedicine*, of which the second edition has just been published.

Natalie Porter is Assistant Professor of Anthropology at the University of Notre Dame, USA. Her ethnographic research examines the production of scientific knowledge and global health interventions for zoonotic disease threats, with a particular focus on avian flu. Her multi-sited research seeks to understand how different actors define zoonoses strategies in their daily interactions with pathogens and their animal hosts and explores how zoonotic threats generate new biological and social relations among nations, institutions, and species. She is currently conducting research on the articulation of wellbeing in dog rescue work, and on the collaborative development of biomedical infrastructures in Cuba and Vietnam.

Ruth Prince is an anthropologist whose recent research focuses on critical global health, biomedicine, state bureaucracies and the public good in East Africa. She is Associate Professor in Medical Anthropology at the University of Oslo, Norway, and principal investigator of the project 'Universal Health Coverage and the Public Good in Africa', a five-year anthropological study funded by a European Research Council Starting Grant, within which she is pursuing research on health insurance markets. Publications relevant to the present volume include a special issue in *Visual Anthropology* with Christos Lynteris, 'Medicine, Anthropology and Photography' (2016); an edited book, *Making* *and Unmaking Public Health in Africa: Ethnographic and Historical Per-spectives*, edited with Rebecca Marsland (Ohio University Press, 2013); and a special issue in *Medical Anthropology Quarterly* titled 'What Is Life Worth? Exploring Biomedical Interventions, Survival, and the Politics of Life' (2012).

Genese Marie Sodikoff is Associate Professor of Anthropology at Rutgers University, USA. Since 1994, her research has focused on Madagascar's political ecology, including the labour politics of biodiversity conservation and cultural and biotic extinction events. Her recent work concerns the impact of zoonotic diseases on Malagasy funerary practices and beliefs in the afterlife. She is the author of *Forest and Labor in Madagascar: From Colonial Concession to Global Biosphere* (Indiana University Press, 2012), and the editor of *The Anthropology of Extinction: Essays on Culture and Species Death* (Indiana University Press, 2011).

Introduction

The anthropology of epidemics

Frédéric Keck, Ann H. Kelly, and Christos Lynteris

Epidemic and pandemic threats contour our contemporary political rationalities and social realities. Emerging and re-emerging infections, from HIV/AIDS to SARS and from Ebola to yellow fever, routinely expose the weakness of our collective systems of disease surveillance and control, fuelling anxieties of future, and increasingly catastrophic, pandemics (Caduff 2015). The 'outbreak narrative' that dominates the contemporary public discourse is propelled by the figure of the commercial aircraft, transporting local contagions across continents (Wald 2008). While the viruses that spill over from wild animals to remote village populations occupy pride of place in these end-of-the-world fantasies (Garret 1994; Preston 1994; see also King 2002; Peckham 2013), today the pathogens that could spark global pandemics might as easily evolve in antimicrobial-rich hospital environments in Europe and the United States (Chandler et al. 2016; Landecker 2016). Epidemics are the dark side of modernisation, medical and political progress; they represent the impossibility of securing the body politic in an ever-more interconnected, technologically advanced and globalised world. Historian Mark Harrison (2016) notes that the term 'pandemic' has been applied to diseases spreading across the globe only since the late nineteenth century, even if other societies have had different ideas about how diseases spread in a given community (which is the Greek meaning of *epidemics*). Responding to, and preparing for, the inevitable and yet unpredictable emergence of new epidemics and pandemics has become a prolific terrain for imagining the future of humanity. Epidemics prompt the question: how and through what mechanisms can we continue to live together?

As a mode of constitution of social life that has been cast anew by recent conceptions of virality, information, and communication, epidemics necessitate not simply the study of the disease itself and the way it affects social relations, but also the study of its modes of anticipation, visualisation, fictionalisation, and materialisation. As a result, what largely began in the mid-1990s as an examination of HIV/AIDS has today come to incorporate the study of a wide range of infectious disease epidemics, with monographs covering cholera, bubonic plague, influenza, Ebola, and dengue. At the same time, the analytic of epidemics has been applied to non-infectious diseases such as obesity or diabetes, as well as to mental illnesses, rendering a general paradigm in medical anthropology. What has made epidemics a particularly rich field of anthropological study is not simply the

DOI: 10.4324/9780429461897-1

multi-layered ethnographic opportunities raised by such phenomena, but primarily the methodological, epistemological, and broader theoretical challenges they pose for the discipline. Drawing together ethnographic insights from a diverse range of sites, histories, and pathogenic trajectories, this volume explores the anthropology of epidemics in a way that frames questions arising from the field as pertinent to the discipline of anthropology as a whole.

Epidemics from anthropological perspectives

Anthropologists have a complicated history with the study of epidemics and their control. Both an obstacle and instrument of imperial expansion, disease outbreaks created the context and justification for policies of segregation, resettlement, quarantine, and population surveillance (Arnold 1993; Hoppe 2003). Epidemics were also an engine of scientific discovery and innovation; key advances in bacteriology and parasitology – for instance, the identification of mosquitoes as disease vectors and the germ theory of disease – developed from the research opportunities afforded by the colonial enterprise (Anderson 2006; Neill 2012). Native and subaltern populations were central to the rise of this new field of scientific inquiry; local traditions, rituals, livelihoods, and domestic spaces were cast as pathogenic reservoirs and as scientific resources for tropical medicine (Lynteris 2016a; Poleykett 2018; Vaughan 1991). Anthropology, a discipline which by the 1920s had come to be defined by a methodological commitment to long-term and immersive fieldwork, promised to render these domains of 'primitive' knowledge and practice visible for scientific interrogation and, in some cases, integration (Schumaker 2001; Tilley 2011).

But rather than being merely another example of anthropology's implication in the colonial domination of indigenous populations, ethnographic engagement with disease control also demonstrates the fragility of the discipline's position within colonialism – and arguably, that of the colonial enterprise itself. Malinowski (1929) famously pleaded for a 'practical anthropology', promoting the study of local systems of law, kinship, and exchange as key units of analysis for colonial development. Native health receives only a passing reference in this influential manifesto, but significantly in terms of the negative consequence of social dislocation introduced by forced labour and rapid urbanisation. At the end of *Primitive Mentality* (1922), a book widely read by colonial officers and literary critics, Lévy-Bruhl showed that mass vaccination failed if local conceptions of epidemics were not considered – a lesson he drew from his visit in the Philippines as an expert for the US colonial government in 1920. The vulnerability of subjugated populations to illness and disease was a key space for critique even when advancing a discourse of the civilising value of colonial occupation. Ethnographic interest in local remedies, healers, therapeutic rituals, and ethnobotanical knowledge reinforced that degree of critical distance, providing anthropologists an empirical line of inquiry that could shed comparative light upon, but not be determined by, Western medicine (Anderson 2006; Feierman and Janzen 1992; Tilley 2011).

Disease outbreaks, however, posed a distinctly more fraught object of ethnographic inquiry and more often than not, colonial medicine (Vaughan 1991). Episodic and exceptional in nature, epidemics are a real-time crisis that compels immediate response (Rosenberg 1992). The devastation disease outbreaks can inflict across populations tends to obviate culturalist interpretations of sickness or health – or at the very least, have made it difficult for local explanatory models to garner the same medical relevance as they have in the context of mental health (Béhague et al. 2008; Kienzler 2008; Kleinman 1992). Social structures and convention retain a certain epidemiological importance, but solely as routes of transmission rather than avenues for cultural exegesis (Trostle 1986). Classical anthropological interrogations of epidemics have therefore either tended to be circumscribed by the immediate demands of containment – for instance, sensitising public health teams to indigenous illness beliefs, identifying problematic customary codes of practice, and enhancing patient-physician trust (Hewlett and Hewlett 2008; Epelboin 2009; Inhorn and Brown 1990; Nichter and Nichter 1996; Janzen 2011).

The double-framing of cultural practice as a vector of disease and as a platform for health promotion links early-twentieth-century tropical hygiene reforms to the health development initiatives implemented by post-colonial states, and finally to latter-day global health security and preparedness programmes (Leach and Scoones 2013; Pigg 1997; Richards 2016). Beyond enhancing the cultural appropriateness of disease containment strategies, anthropological attention to local explanations and experiences of epidemic events provided a critical space to interrogate the differing social impacts of outbreak response and the forms of social exclusion, blame, and panic these interventions surface (Baer et al. 2003; Lindenbaum 2001). Arguably, then, this line of anthropological inquiry is to understand epidemics as *plagues* – what Herring and Swedlund (2010) characterise by 'cycles of shame and blame, stigmatizing discourses, isolation of the sick' (2010: 4–5). Not merely epidemiological trends, but 'critical events', outbreaks have the capacity to reorder social relations (Das 1995) and generate new subjectivities (Lynteris 2014), precipitating not only physical suffering but moral crises that can upend collective modes of existence (Alcabes 2009; Lindenbaum 1979).

The outbreak of HIV/AIDS shifted and amplified the dimensions of anthropological engagement with epidemics. For many anthropologists, the scale of the outbreak exposed the shortcomings of conventional ethnographic emphasis on disease as symbolic practice detached from history and political-economic context (Scheper-Hughes and Lock 1986). On the one hand, the stigma associated with the disease problematised a straightforwardly culturalist approach that failed to denounce extreme acts of public health negligence (Schoepf 2001). On the other hand, the effectiveness of anti-retroviral treatment obviated social-behavioural risk, as epidemic control came to hinge upon the distribution of life-saving pharmaceuticals (Brandt 2013; Hardon and Dilger 2011). Anthropological attention focused on the biopolitics of therapeutic access and the structural inequities that underpinned the vast discrepancies in health outcomes between and within populations (Farmer 2004; Fassin 2007; Lock and Nguyen 2010). Bearing witness to the suffering visited upon infected individuals by the global political economy, anthropological work was put to the service of global health advocacy and activism (Robbins 2004; Biehl and Petryna 2013).

In addition to providing 'empirical lanterns' to individual and social suffering (Biehl 2016; Das et al. 2001), anthropologists have interrogated the discursive configuration of HIV/AIDS within an emerging regime of biosecurity (Caduff 2014; Collier et al. 2004). In 2000, the United Nations Security Council took the unprecedented step of declaring the HIV/AIDS epidemic a threat to international security in Africa. While justified by the global health community as means to garner international attention to the crisis, inscribing infectious disease within the language of danger and risk effectively normalised techniques and administrative practices that cast infected individuals as a form of national threat (Elbe 2008). The militarisation of public health reached an apotheosis in the wake of 9/11, whereby preparing for emerging disease became a central arm in the pre-emptive war against terror (Cooper 2006; Masco 2014). Illuminating the geopolitical contours and consequences of biosecurity, anthropologists have demonstrated how epidemics, or rather their perennial imminent threat, provide the pretext for the extension of governmental power across all forms of life and manner of living (Caduff 2014). That scholarship also shows how the radical expansion of strategies of containment ultimately works to narrow the scope of public health practice, giving precedence to the projected risks posed by imagined catastrophic contagious events rather than to the everyday social inequalities and global inequities that determine who becomes infected in the first place (Fee and Brown 2001; Lachenal 2015).

Epidemics, Charles Rosenberg suggests, are described as terrifying phenomena that 'create an imperative need for understanding. Such explanatory efforts necessarily reflect a particular generation's cultural and intellectual assumptions, its repertoire of available tools' (1992: 34). In bringing together anthropological engagements with the field of epidemics, this volume seeks to develop tools to examine these phenomena and their wider social impact. Three thematic threads link the chapters of this book: the study of zoonotic disease or interspecies transmission of pathogens, the infrastructural and material aspects of epidemics, and counter-epidemic intervention. This is not because these are the only themes explored and examined by anthropologists interested in epidemic disease today, but because we believe that it is on the lines of these themes where the anthropological study of epidemics is producing analytical insights and unsettlements most relevant to anthropological thinking as a whole. Rather than being yet another collection of disease ethnographies, this volume aspires to bring epidemics to the forefront of anthropological debate, as an exemplary arena for social scientific study and analysis.

Interspecies transmission and zoonotic pathogens

The idea of zoonosis, or the infection of humans by diseases carried by animals, is a distinctly modern medical notion. Initially applied to rabies but acquiring its full semantic and epistemic force in relation to plague in the first decades of the twentieth century, zoonosis is today widely recognised as one of the most complex and pressing epidemiological questions. Anthropological interest in zoonosis has flourished in the past five years. Whereas anthropologists have long studied diseases of zoonotic origin, such as HIV/AIDS, it is only recently that these are studied *as zoonoses*, with anthropological focus placed on animal to human infection (Keck and Lynteris 2018). This turn has been catalysed by the importance of zoonosis for the broader paradigm shift in virology and bacteriology known by the name of Emerging Infectious Disease: the idea that pathogens hitherto only carried by non-human animals are able to mutate and 'spill over' to humans, causing great mortality in populations never exposed to them before (King 2002; Quammen 2012). Rather than this remaining a scientific arcanum, increased media coverage of the zoonotic aspects of epidemic like SARS, influenza, and Ebola, coupled with cinematographic configurations of animals as the source of killer viruses threatening humanity with extinction (Ostherr 2005), have placed zoonosis well into the public eye.

Anthropologists have thus tried to negotiate a particularly entangled situation. First, by critically engaging with epistemological frameworks of zoonosis and disease emergence as these are developed in scientific communities. Second, by accounting for the public appeal and spectacle of zoonosis, as a source of existential risk, and the way this is used to generate or direct global health policy. And third, by understanding both historically and ethnographically the social aspects and dynamics of animal to human infection, and the impact of zoonosis as a scientific doctrine and a popular imaginary on the ground. From explanatory model to inductive method to charismatic prophesy, zoonosis is quickly developing into a cornerstone social fact of twenty-first-century globalised societies.

A key aspect in the anthropological examination of zoonosis, and one that has particular significance regarding anthropological debates outside the confines of medical anthropology, regards the broader field of interspecies relations. In the last twenty years, social anthropology has undergone what has been called an 'ontological turn', which should be understood in two ways. First, it refers to a new gaze on non-human animals, which is not caught up in the symbolic webs of culture but is rather attentive to the interactions and entanglements between co-evolving species. In this new mode of anthropological description, animals are not considered as passive carriers of long-term human symbols but rather as actors in unstable and vulnerable networks of co-existence. Second, the ontological turn leads ethnographers to take seriously the claims of societies that attribute actions to animals, and brings them in a conversation with other commitments about animal agency. Notions of local knowledge taken from ethno-zoology are thus reactivated in the wake of the challenges raised by zoonoses, raising new questions on the modes of agency of pathogens transmitted from animals to humans. These two meanings of the ontological turn in social anthropology rephrase the general idea, common in evolutionary biology, that humans, animals, and microbes co-evolve in bounded ecosystems, but in a way that pays attention to the local configurations of these forms of interaction and to the global effects of the transgression of what appears as ecological boundaries by 'spillover events'. The transmission of tuberculosis between humans and elephants in Southeast Asia as a 'reverse zoonosis' following the rise of ecological tourism (Lainé 2018), or the enigmas of the transmission of MERS-CoV between camels and humans in the Arab Peninsula without a bat reservoir after the development of international camel racing (Cabalion et al. 2018), have thus led to investigations of interspecies entanglements at the local and global levels.

These theoretical and political questions within the debates of anthropology have met with interdisciplinary collaborations at the level of global health. Indeed, veterinarians and ecologists are increasingly required to collaborate with microbiologists and epidemiologists to provide knowledge on the transmission of pathogens from animals to humans and thus anticipate the emergence of zoonotic pathogens. The efforts to manage the ontological complexity of pathogenic circulations, labelled under the term 'One Health', operate across radically uneven political landscapes, and in their appeals to ecological holism they can obviate and exacerbate pre-existing vulnerabilities between species and among humans (Craddock and Hinchliffee 2015). They also provide a framework in which information on pathogenic mutations is standardised, mutualised, and exchanged through shared databases, which tends to evacuate the diversity of professional habits in collecting materials from animals (Fortané and Keck 2015).

The 'One Health' initiative can thus be described as an attempt to produce purified information from the impure circulation of animals across the globe. Indeed, scientific frameworks of zoonotic infection have singled out animals alongside an 'included' versus 'rogue' binary (Fairhead 2018b). Dating back to the identification in colonial India of the rat as the main source of bubonic plague (Evans 2018), the idea of rogue zoonotic sources has been tied to notions of invisibility which, while predating bacteriology, became a key aspect of epidemiology as a result of Pasteurian emphasis on bacterial attenuation and recrudescence (Lynteris 2017a, Lynteris in print; Mendhelson 2002. In the age of 'emergence', colonial strategies of sliding scales of medical blame, involving both native subjects and animal species (Evans 2018), continue to inform epidemiological practice. Fairhead (2018b) thus argues that in the context of the Ebola epidemic in West Africa, rogue status shifted according to context from the virus, to the bat, to bushmeat hunters, to the sick themselves. What, however, differentiates zoonotic framings in the age of emergence from those in the time of what we may call high-modern epidemiology (roughly 1870s–1970s) is that 'Rogues connote not only the age-old threat that the excluded pose to power, but also its new emergent uknowability' (Fairhead 2018b: 175). Whereas high-modern epidemiology relied on a doctrine of progress, accompanied by one of a hygienic utopia, envisioned in terms of an efficient separation of humans from pathogens and the animals that carry them, the age of emergence is pervaded by a pessimistic outlook of the world, that necessitates new forms of power and knowledge for the maintenance of human mastery over human/non-human relations (Lynteris 2017b). This is a state of affairs that is evident in the ways zoonosis is being visualised both in scientific and popular representations of disease and infection.

Growing historical and anthropological interest in the way epidemics are visualised has led to studies that go beyond the usual illustrative or representational focus on epidemic images. Seen as a process that contributes but also challenges epistemological and political aspects of epidemics, visualisation is thus becoming a new terrain of medical anthropological research. Studies of what Lynteris has coined 'epidemic photography' (2016c) have led to a closer understanding of the way in which photography has been used to render epidemics intelligible and actionable: from uses of photography in mapping epidemic terrains (Engelmann 2018) and the importance of photographic practices in the rise of colonial regimes of epidemiological knowledge (Poleykett 2017) to the photographic configuration of live animal or so-called 'wet markets' in China as the ground zero of the 'next pandemic' (Lynteris 2016c). More than simply being a permutation of medical photography, epidemic photography captures the past, present, and future of epidemic events and processes, drawing out an epidemic potentiality across social existence. Epidemic photography does not simply render the causes, victims, or drivers of epidemics visible. Rather, it forges a powerful dialectic between visibility and invisibility. Contra the ontological focus of proponents of the 'bacteriological revolution' (Latour 1993; Cunningham 1992), it is through their constant visualisation (rather than in spite of it) that infectious diseases have remained at what, following Smith (2013), we can call the edge of scientific sight; a state of constant epistemological unsettlement that has been further enhanced by what Nicholas King (2004) has described as the emergence of infectious disease emergence frameworks.

In the present volume, Lynteris examines how photography operates after the end of an epidemic outbreak so as to foster a suspension of epidemiological certainties that often solidify in response to infectious disease in the course of outbreaks. He examines the photographic output of the Chinese-Russian plague expedition to South Siberia and Mongolia, led by Wu Liande and Danilo Zabolotny, following the end of the devastating pneumonic plague epidemic in Manchuria in 1911. The photographs produced and collected by Wu neither confirmed nor disavowed his hitherto held belief in the implication of marmots in the spread of plague. Instead they opened up a space of doubt and uncertainty that remains invisible in textual records, which, by contrast, stress Wu's conversion into the idea that marmots had nothing to do with the disease. In its verbal silence, epidemic photography thus allows us a closer, phenomenological view of scientific research, its epistemological lacunas and suspensions, in a space where scientific imagination can be deployed and developed.

On the other hand, literary and cultural studies scholars (Boluk and Lenz 2010; Gomel 2000; Ostherr 2005; Schweitzer 2018; Wald 2008) have showed that fictional accounts (films, TV programmes, paperbacks, videogames) of the 'next pandemic' as an event posing an existential risk to humanity give rise to imaginaries of ends of the world. Following Deborah Danowski and Eduardo Viveiros de Castro (2016), these should be seen not simply as apocalyptic fantasies, but as normative scripts about the relation between humankind and the world which both generate and unsettle visions of mastery over human/non-human relations

(Lynteris 2017b). Imaginaries of viruses as mutants and as enemies mobilise different regimes of norms and ontologies of human–animal relations (Keck 2015). This visual culture has had a pronounced applied aspect as regards epidemic control. Riding the wave of zombie visual culture, and the image of the epidemiologist as a culture hero promoted by films on pandemic catastrophe (Lynteris 2016b), the US CDC's 2011 pandemic preparedness campaign mobilised popular fascination with the 'undead' in what has been hailed as the most successful communication stint of the agency (Fraustino and Ma 2015; Halabi et al. 2013; Kruvand and Silver 2013): *Preparedness 101: Zombie Pandemic* (Silver 2011).

Such collusion between public health agencies and the cultural industry may be said to contribute to what Briggs (2017) has identified as communicative inequities, in the context of epidemics and epidemic threats. The idea of communicative inequity is a powerful anthropological tool that underlines the ways in which, beyond global health fantasies and fetishisations of data sharing, on the actual ground what counts as meaningful and actionable evidence, how information is distributed, and the way this accrues value depend on pervasive racial, gender, and class hierarchies. Whether these are photographs, maps, or diagrams, images and their visual economy play a key role in epidemic communication not only in terms of educating and convincing, but, more importantly, as a way of defining and policing what counts as knowledge and what can be discounted as rumour, stories, or anecdote. From a visual anthropological perspective, this clearly points out the fact that images of epidemics and zoonoses are not mere representations of infectious diseases and their social impact, but rather actants in a broader political economic arena of power and knowledge.

Infrastructures and materialities

The inequities that Briggs tracks through outbreak narratives, biosecurity discussions, scientific explanations, and public health dialogue gives semiotic depth to the 'social machinery of oppression' that preoccupies anthropological accounts of HIV/AIDS (Farmer 2004: 312). A key empirical advantage of a linguistic purview on epidemics is the attention it draws to pragmatic practices of exchange – the flows of knowledge, circulation of information, and communicative systems – that stabilise a crisis into an object of intervention and transform populations into compliant subjects or sites of resistance (Briggs 2011; see also Leach and Tadros 2014). Recent anthropological interest in urban infrastructure develops this ethnographic concern with the systems that enable circulation, exploring the intersections of material and immaterial, visible and invisible boundaries that contour the operations of social, economic, and political life (e.g. De Boeck 2015; Lockrem and Lugo 2015; Simone 2004). This scholarship provides an exceptionally fertile ground for conceptualising epidemics not only as objects of public health and scientific concern, but also as dynamic fields of pathogenicity, moving between material surfaces, objects, and human and non-human bodies.

Disease ecologists have developed a rich vocabulary to articulate the heterogeneous pathogenic interaction that drives epidemics. Terms like 'hot spot' and 'viral chatter' capture the spatial and temporal contingencies that can lead to the emergence of a disease and its establishment in a human population (e.g. DeGroote et al. 2008; Johnson et al. 2010; Wolfe 2011). Transmission, this work teaches us, is never simply the matter of a single moment or point of contact, but rather is varied and disproportionate, amplified through particular characteristics of individuals, populations, and environments or, for instance, in the case of the Broad Street Pumps, contaminated things (Lloyd-Smith et al. 2005). Taking their ethnographic cue for this relational approach to viral space, anthropologists have shifted their attention to the experiences and understanding of disease to the material practices and proximities of everyday life that prompt infection (Brown and Kelly 2014; Singer 2017; see also Fontein 2011). 'Infrastructural-thinking' has allowed a transgressive ethnographic approach. On one hand, attending to the convergences of pathogenic potential collapses formally distinct public health (and to a certain degree, anthropological) domains of the household, the hospital, the farm, the market, and the forest. On the other, understanding the social and political conditions that occasion those convergences demands a historically nuanced understanding of the entanglements – between for instance, colonial-era plantations, village farms, and a population of migrating bats, or between farms and markets of live chickens – that persist in a shared landscape. In contrast to an 'outbreak timeline', these anthropological accounts do not reconstruct a single route of infection, but rather excavate a latent pathogenic milieu.

In her chapter in this volume, Genese Marie Sodikoff explores rat burrows in Madagascar as a complex non-human infrastructure implicated in seasonal outbreaks of plague on the island. What does it mean to examine the recurring outbreaks of human plague on the island through the lens of 'multispecies, multilayered infrastructure[s] of *Y. pestis*'? Sodikoff argues that what makes rat burrows particularly important is that they do not simply connect humans with the natural reservoir of the bacterium in that region (the rat), but that they do so by means of an entanglement with human cadavers and their resting places. Whether this occurs in reality or only in the epidemiological imagination, the way in which the interlinkage of living rat infrastructures and infrastructures of human death is invested as catalytic for the maintenance and periodic return of plague back to the living is of key importance for social life in the plague-affected areas of Madagascar: 'by forging imagined routes between rats and buried kin, [burrow systems] also link marginalised rural communities to the state in undesirable ways, sustaining a historical resistance to biomedical authority'.

Indeed, a key focus-point of anthropological attention to the infrastructure of epidemics is technologies and materiality of response. In their examination of the techniques of epidemic control, Lynteris and Poleykett (2018) have argued that 'as anthropologists, we need to take seriously the self-positioning of epidemic control as technologically advanced, and consider the contemporary entanglement between counter-epidemic technologies of different historical provenance on the ethnographic ground'. If, as Wolf and Hall (2018) have shown, preparedness 'organizes people around specific emergency infrastructures and communication routines', regimes of exception employed with increasing ease in response to outbreaks rely on the spatial organisation of epidemic spaces in terms of infectiously inflected zones (see also Nading 2017).

While radically out of step with the humanitarian ethic of global health, there is a seductive resonance between pre-bacteriological public health practice and contemporary biosecurity preoccupations with disease emergence. Anthropological attention is needed, then, to the shifting material forms attendant not only to the control of epidemics but to the material production of anticipatory knowledge related to practical interventions in the field. Disease ecology is a complex mediation between standardised controls in a laboratory setting and local conditions in the field (Anderson 2004; Kelly and Lezaun 2017; Lezaun and Montgomery 2015). The distributed quality of epidemiological credibility depends on an assortment of practices and techniques, including reference materials, good laboratory practice (GLP) protocols, quality control panels, training, procurement regulations, and clinical algorithms.

But further ethnographic insight is needed into the local forms of biosecurity practice and containment upon which livelihoods depend. Natalie Porter's chapter in this volume gives ethnographic contour to the everyday organisation and disruption of containment by examining the stories of transnational migration and return among export labour migrants from Bac Giang province in rural northern Vietnam. She demonstrates how the infusion of foreign capital in rural economies transforms poultry production patterns in ways that engender new disease vulnerabilities for animals and humans. New forms of casual labour arising from a fragile, but increasingly transnational, entrepreneurialism upend kin-based systems of land management and livestock care upon which the health of animals depend. Biosecurity in this context is a feature of social stability; the capricious arrival and departure of migrant kin, cascading obligations, and expectations of financial gain, took families away from their flocks or lead them to compromise standards of poultry containment (see also Porter 2013). The examples Porter draws of the embedded sociality of epidemic control unsettles dominant narratives of that focus on urbanisation and spillover, by attending to the complex aspirations, capacities, and investments of increasingly mobile, and increasingly wealthy, rural populations.

Knowing epidemics, in other words, poses a distinct challenge concerning the relationship between credibility, anticipation, and efficacy: in contexts of primary health care, humanitarian intervention, and epidemiological research, the issue is not only how credible scientific results are produced, but what can be done with them, and by whom.

Intervention and collaboration

Intervention in epidemics, in the form of containment and control, has been a subject of intensive study by historians of medicine like Anderson (2006), David Arnold (1993), Alison Bashford (2014), Mark Harrison (2012), and others. Stressing the colonial genealogy of contemporary counter-epidemic interventions, more recently anthropologists have drawn attention to epistemic lacunas and unsettlements in colonial approaches of epidemic diseases. Underlining that the production of epidemiological knowledge and forms of population control has been intricately intertwined, they have shown that colonial responses to epidemics relied on frameworks of pathogenic tropicality. Importantly, these studies can help us understand key but misrecognised aspects of contemporary forms of epidemiological knowledge and practice. To give but one example, if Pasteurian concerns with hygienic burials of plague victims in Madagascar in the 1920s (Poleykett 2018; Sodikoff this volume) anticipate anxieties over 'traditional' burials during the Ebola epidemic in West Africa in 2014–15, this should not be seen as simply a colonial relic, but rather as part of persistence of the infectious corpse as an epistemic object of modern epidemiology and as a locus of public health intervention (a double 'sliding object' in this sense) that continues to generate fear, concern, research, and policy today (Lynteris and Evans 2018; Fairhead 2018a).

The biosecurity agenda provides an important context for the most recent turn in the anthropology of epidemics: the call for their inclusion in emergency outbreak response (WHO 2018; DFID-Wellcome 2018). What Stellmach and colleagues characterise as a 'renewed recognition of the need to understand social pathways of disease transmission and barriers to care' follows on the heels of the 2014–16 Ebola outbreak, for which the lack of community engagement and unilateral disregard of local practices were regarded as chief amongst the reasons for the exacerbation of crisis (Stellmach et al. 2018: 1; WHO 2015). Building upon the insights of work on HIV/AIDS and biosecurity, anthropologists pointed to the determining role of entrenched poverty in epidemic amplification (e.g. Farmer 2016; Wilkinson and Leach 2015) and the profound health inequities attendant to the sensationalism of the emergency response (Kelly and Marí-Sáez 2018; Lachenal 2014; Nuñes 2016). However, the visibility and presumed epidemiological relevance of a particular set of 'cultural traditions'– for instance, those involving burial, secret societies, healers, and witchcraft – provided a fulcrum for anthropological engagement with the Ebola response (Martineau et al. 2017; Sams and Desclaux 2017). 'Cultural practice' provided an epistemic common ground for anthropologists, policy makers, and public health professionals operating under conditions of radical uncertainty (Bolten and Sheper 2017).

Rather than this being a recent development, or one restricted to anthropologists, the relapse to ethnographically procured cultural certainties in the light of biological uncertainty has showed itself a constitutive element of epidemiology since its emergence as a discipline (Lynteris 2016a). Indeed, it may be claimed that having historically emerged in tandem within shared institutional and ideological frameworks, anthropology and epidemiology have much more in common than their current self-presentation may allow us to believe. Key to both disciplines has been the notion of contagion, a pre-epidemiological idea that with the rise of bacteriology and the systematisation of the study of disease transmission accrued scientific value by the end of the nineteenth century (Harrison 2012; Wald 2008). At the same time that contagion was being transformed through laboratory science and statistics, it formed the basis for understanding social processes in foundational anthropological and sociological works by James Frazer, Gustave

Le Bon, and Gabriel Tarde (Lynteris and Evans 2018; Rosental 2011; Sampson 2012; Wald 2008). Indeed, ideas of social contagion are still prevalent today not only in anthropology (e.g. Grøn and Meinert 2017) but across Western societies where it and its synecdoches (virality being the most prevalent) are no longer simply a metaphor for economic crises, riots, terrorism, or social media trends (Magnusson and Zalloua 2012), but as 'a cause-effect relation *literally* underlining' such phenomena (Lynteris and Evans 2018: 4). In other words, contagion is conceived as both an anthropological universal (e.g. Caprara 1998) and as 'the dominant modality through which to describe that which might simultaneously realize and destroy the social' (Lynteris and Evans 2018: 7). Contagion, as Lorenzo Servitje and Kari Nixon playfully put it, 'is endemic to our contemporary culture' (2016: 1).

In his chapter for this volume, Carlo Caduff thus asks: 'What makes a disease communicable in our culture of media?' Arguing that 'the mass media has found in the idea of the next pandemic an ideal opportunity to corroborate its own discursive problematic', Caduff explores the idea of epidemic seriality: 'At its root, the world of preparedness entails a political form attuned to economies of mass production. It thrives on serial figures that are proliferating in technomediated milieus'. The demand of the serialisation ad nauseam which forms the backbone of the culture industry is thus shown to be linked to forms of pleasure associated with the 'promise of making repetition a moment of renewal'. Drawing on the affinities between global health and capitalist mentalities through the mythic 'demand to consider what's next' (the next pandemic, in epidemiology, the next deal in the market, the next show in mass culture), Caduff expands Brian Massumi's turn from biopower to ontopower (2015), so as to show that what he calls the 'serialisation of serialisation' generates a temporality with no closure in sight. Through the generation of 'provisional ends' 'the next unfolds and reinvents itself by virtue of a constitutive reiterative openness that never brings rest to the now'.

Andrew Lakoff, in his chapter for this volume, asks a different question, derived from Ian Hacking's historical ontology: 'What is an epidemic emergency?'. The problem he raises is how epidemics are declared to start and end, and how these official classifications make them real. In the series of continuous mutations and transmissions of pathogens, public institutions frame an epidemic as a significant course of event, that also gives rise to meaningful narratives in the media. Taking Ebola and Zika as two examples of recent epidemic emergencies, Lakoff shows that controversies were raised precisely on when epidemics started and ended to justify public health interventions. Preparedness, concludes Lakoff, is more than a constant state of readiness to the continuous mutations of microbes: it is a measurable condition, requiring methods of testing and sets of standards.

In their chapter, Keck and Lachenal add another element to Caduff and Lakoff's diagnoses of preparedness. Through a review of different forms of simulations of epidemics in Asia and Africa they explore, by means of the anthropology of ritual, how exercises and drills mobilise humans, animals, and artefacts to produce the imaginary of the epidemic to come, be they organised in a closed room with computers or in the public space with actors. Critics of exercises are always raised in terms of the realism of the simulation, because what counts in the exercise is the engagement of actors in the reality of the epidemic to come. Simulation, Keck and Lachenal conclude, has become a technique of government in neo-liberal societies because individuals and states are assessed on their capacity to engage in a test which produces its own forms of reality.

In these tests of social reality provided by epidemic outbreaks, anthropologists are supposed to engage themselves, because they are required to define the formats of the tests and to include a wider range of actors. Indeed, the post-Ebola global health landscape offers exciting opportunities for collaborative engagement. Arguably for the first time, anthropologists are being actively sought – as part of institutional policy – to participate on national and international decision-making bodies for epidemic preparedness. Though perhaps remarkable considering the discipline's penchant for long-term immersion in the field, anthropologists are currently being cast as facilitators in the rapid production and uptake of knowledge, the fast-tracking of community outreach, and the real-time integration of behavioural and epidemiological insights (Abramowitz et al. 2018). The question for anthropologists is the extent to which these will frustrate or catalyse methodological innovations and conceptual advances for the discipline. If the hallmark of an anthropology of HIV/AIDS was a 'historically deep and geographically broad analysis' (Farmer 2004: 309) – an interpretive frame that would evidence the role and reach of institutionalised racism – the anthropological project currently envisioned for epidemic emergencies is one suited for the accelerated deployment interventions; we are being brought into the fold to corroborate and extend the forms of counting that characterise both epidemiology and the broader global health project (Adams 2016).

There is tremendous potential here to make anthropology count for policy and moreover to make its methodology available for the populations we study; anthropologists working within the field of humanitarianism have repeatedly shown how in urgent situations local staff have profound ethnographic potential (see Allen and Schomerus 2008). However, if the critique of structural violence remains a theoretical framework and moral imperative for anthropology, its normative orientation within epidemic preparedness and emergency epidemic remains somewhat uncertain. The Ebola outbreak, for instance, provides examples of what can be occluded by a focus on contagion in contrast to the configurations of power and knowledge epidemics put in motion. It was a public health disaster but also a research opportunity: vaccines that had been conceived in the context of a post-9/11 biosecurity agenda were rapidly developed in emergency clinical trials. The intense scramble for Ebola cases that began following the wane of the outbreak, shows how humanitarian crises have also become an engine for capital (Erikson 2015; Kelly 2018; see also Sunder Rajan 2006). There is a concern that the operational demands of outbreak control might blunt the critical force of ethnographic accounts, particularly with regards to how epidemics are constructed as matters of public health, humanitarian, and biosecurity problems (Stellmach 2013). Vinh-Kim Nguyen's chapter in this volume is a testimony of the engagement of a group of anthropologists in the aftermath of the Ebola crisis. Noting that the moral question for anthropologists is that of the discrepancy of speed between different modes of intervention in the temporality of the crisis, he shows that the problem of how to connect viruses at different speeds of evolution is also raised by molecular epidemiology at the level of the infrastructure. The interspecies zone, concludes Nguyen, is a space where these different speeds can be negotiated to avoid violent confrontation because no species barrier or disciplinary boundary defines in advance the limits of contagion and collaboration.

Death – particularly on the scale of epidemics – tends to short-circuit processes of signification: to die from infectious disease is in many ways to meet an unspeakable end. An end, moreover, that in the Western imaginary is metonymically associated, at least since Thucydides' narrative of the 'plague' of Athens, with societal collapse (Lynteris and Evans 2018). Empirically unfounded and indeed covering up much more complex sociological and historical responses to disease outbreaks (Cohn 2018), the idea that epidemics dissolve social ties, lead to individualistic behaviour, and ultimately end up in a generalised state of anomy, forms part of distinctly naturalist definitions of human sociality: as a precarious state of 'culture' constantly threatened by instantaneous collapse into 'nature'. More often than not, collaboration and its funding depend precisely on this sociological fantasy, which anthropologists are called to critique and demonstrate its impact on the ground.

At the same time as relying on and reproducing meta-narratives about humanity, counter-epidemic interventions also interpellate specific 'publics'. In her chapter in this volume, Ruth Prince examines how 'through flows of global funding and transnational interventions', some groups or populations have accrued 'social visibility and political traction while others faded into the background'. Introducing the term 'pandemic publics' so as 'to draw attention to the interplay of visibility and presentation, voice, and audience in the process by which particular collectives are brought into being over the course of an epidemic', Prince stresses that in the case of HIV/AIDS in Kisumu, Kenya, any given group's success in the competition for resources made available by NGOs and other organisations in the midst of the epidemic depended on 'their ability to present themselves in terms that global health organisations and actors could understand'. The drive to make themselves visible in a way that stresses 'their belonging to and identification with "the community"', while simultaneously 'striving to differentiate themselves as responsible actors in, rather than as targets of, development' reproduced 'lines of social and moral distinction' in relation to the disease (cf Esposito 2011). And, at the same time, Prince argues, it also fostered a depoliticisation of health care, 'encouraging individuals and groups to make claims based on needs rather than entitlements, to NGOs rather than to their elected governments and to the state'.

Unfolding thus in an intellectual, institutional, and economic environment defined by emergency and discourses of existential risk, the anthropology of epidemics faces the challenge of two extremes: on the one hand, uncritical engagement and collaboration in the name of human lives, and on the other hand, critical distancing and self-guarded isolation in the name of knowledge. For those who tread the middle path of critical engagement or engaged critique, the challenge is not only dealing with offended biologists or suspicious anthropologists, but of envisioning what a critical epidemiology may be, what could be its aims, programme, and principles. In her chapter in this volume, Hannah Brown draws on ethnographic experience with two epidemics (HIV in East Africa and Ebola in West Africa) in order to see how 'models of complexity in social sciences and biomedicine' interact in the context of managing outbreaks of infectious diseases. On the one hand, Brown argues, the aim of anthropology is 'to capture nuance and complexity, rendering visible these dimensions of social life to those who read their work'. On the other hand, public health, especially when disease control is concerned, 'often centres on activities that aim to simplify complexity'. So whereas key plague scientists of zoonotic diseases may admit that, as regards the disease ecology of the latter, we are in a state of 'epistemological entropy' (Kosoy 2013), when it comes to controlling such diseases in the context of an emergency 'straightforward guidelines' aimed 'to help people navigate through complex worlds' become necessary. Yet Brown argues that this is not simply a story of anthropological complexity versus epidemic-control simplicity. Indeed, what is more pressing is the negotiation of different forms of complexity in the two collaborating fields. Focused on risk-aversion, public health professionals 'see complexity [as] a problem to be dealt with primarily though documentation, organisation, and planning'. By contrast, anthropologists recognise that in spite of all their immersive ethnographic engagement there is a level of complexity (or indeed several of them) that cannot be known but which remains as it were at the edge of ethnographic sight. Rather than assuming the two approaches of complexity are simply antithetical, Brown proposes a dialogical model according to which anthropological attention to the ways in which responses to epidemics unfold on the ground, and the way in which ethnography is attuned to unexpected dimensions of responses to epidemics constitute important sites at which anthropological work can contribute within outbreak response and public health interventions more widely.

***

This volume explores the contemporary problem epidemics pose for anthropologists as an object of study and engagement. What has made epidemics a particularly rich field of anthropological study is not simply the multi-layered ethnographic opportunities raised by such phenomena but primarily the methodological, epistemological, ethical, and broader theoretical challenges they pose for the discipline. Following from previous efforts to consider epidemics as an idea (Herring and Swedlund 2010: 2), contributors consider the modes of relationality the epidemic brings to light. As a mode of constitution of social life that has been cast anew by recent conceptions of virality, information, and communication, epidemics necessitate not simply the study of the disease itself but the way it configures social relations. If terms like spillover, hotspot, sentinel, or emergence have been used to capture that contingent, latent, and recursive capacity of epidemics, anthropological accounts can describe this bio-communicability whose tempos and scales challenge the ways we imagine both social life and the publics of public health (Briggs 2011; Brown and Kelly 2014; Keck and Lakoff 2015).

Moreover, contributors explore the epistemic contours of epidemics. Characterised by their potential to surprise and elude our systems of knowledge, outbreaks are 'black swan events'demanding speculative and creative modes of attention, ones that trouble the conventional epistemic contours of social science intelligence (Lakoff 2010). How epidemics are brought into view, what is rendered visible and invisible, requires the study not only of the epidemiological event but the study of its modes of anticipation, visualisation, fictionalisation, and materialisation that render it intelligible and amenable to intervention (Löwy 2010).

Finally, contributors hope to consider the moral questions epidemics pose for the discipline: how do anthropologists balance the corroborative potential and critical demands of ethnographic practice within the investigation of epidemic crises (Bornstein and Redfield 2010); Benton 2015)? Outbreaks are also occasions when global concerns impinge on matters of state, reconstituting the domains of government and citizenship (Lowe 2017; Mitropoulos 2012) and causing deadly frictions between scientific rationalities, public health norms, and cultural processes (Hinchliffe and Ward 2014; Keck 2008; Tsing 2004). Like other catastrophic events, outbreaks have the capacity to exacerbate existing social tensions and create new ones to trigger both administrative collapse and political change (e.g. Choy 2005; Fortun 2009).

This edited volume aspires to be the first comprehensive collection of papers on the anthropology of epidemics, incorporating key theoretical perspectives and overarching questions which make the particular subject pertinent not only to medical anthropology but to the discipline as a whole, setting anthropology at the forefront of social scientific examination of epidemics today.

Acknowledgements

Research by Christos Lynteris leading to this chapter was funded by a European Research Council Starting Grant under the European Union's Seventh Framework Programme/ERC grant agreement no 336564 for the project Visual Representations of the Third Plague Pandemic (University of St Andrews). Ann H. Kelly's contribution was supported by the U.K. Economic and Social Research Council Urgency Research Grant Scheme (grant no. ES/M009203/1).

References

Abramowitz, Sharon A., David B. Hipgrave, Alison Witchard, and David L. Heymann 'Lessons from The West Africa Ebola epidemic: A systematic review of epidemiological and social and behavioral science research priorities', *Journal of Infectious Diseases* (2018) accepted manuscript. https://academic.oup.com/jid/advance-article/doi/10.1093/infdis/jiy387/5043310

Adams, Vincanne *Metrics: What Counts in Global Health* (Durham, NC: Duke University Press, 2016).

Alcabes, Philip *Dread: How Fear and Fantasy Have Fueled Epidemics from the Black Death to Avian Flu* (New York: Public Affairs, 2009).

Allen, Tim, and Mareike Schomerus *Complex Emergencies and Humanitarian Responses* (London: University of London, 2008).

Anderson, Warwick 'Natural histories of infectious disease: Ecological vision in twentieth-century Biomedical Science', *Osiris* 19 (2004), 39–61.

Anderson, Warwick *Colonial Pathologies: American Tropical Medicine, Race, and Hygiene in the Philippines* (Durham, NC: Duke University Press, 2006).

Arnold, David *Colonizing the Body: State Medicine and Epidemic Disease in Nineteenth-Century India* (Berkeley, CA: The University of California Press, 1993).

Baer, Hans A., Merrill Singer, and Ida Susser *Medical Anthropology and the World System* (Westport, CT: Greenwood Publishing Group, 2003).

Bashford, Alison *Imperial Hygiene. A Critical History of Colonialism, Nationalism and Public Health* (London: Palgrave Macmillan, 2014).

Béhague, Dominique Pareja, Helen Gonçalves, and Cesar Gomes Victora 'Anthropology and epidemiology: Learning epistemological lessons through a collaborative venture', *Ciencia & saude coletiva* 13 (6) (2008), 1701–1710.

Benton, Adia. *HIV Exceptionalism: Development Through Disease in Sierra Leone* (Minneapolis: Minnesota University Press, 2015).

Biehl, João 'Theorizing global health', *Medicine Anthropology Theory* 3 (2) (2016), 127–142.

Biehl, João, and Adriana Petryna *When People Come First* (Princeton, NJ: Princeton University Press, 2013).

Bolten, Catherine, and Susan Shepler 'Producing Ebola: Creating knowledge in and about an epidemic', *Anthropology Quarterly* 90 (2) (2017), 349–368.

Boluk, Stephanie and Wylie Lenz 'Infection, media, and capitalism: From early modern plagues to postmodern zombies', *Journal for Early Modern Cultural Studies* 10 (2) (2010), 126–147.

Bornstein, Erica, and Peter Redfield 'An introduction to the anthropology of humanitarianism', In Peter Redfield, and Erica Bornstein (eds.), *Forces of Compassion: Humanitarianism Between Ethics and Politics*, pp. 3–30 (Sante Fe: School for Advanced Research Press, 2010).

Brandt, Allan M. 'How AIDS invented global health', *New England Journal of Medicine* 368 (23) (2013), 2149–2152.

Briggs, Charles, L. 'Communicating biosecurity', *Medical Anthropology* 30 (2011), 6–29.

Briggs, Charles L. 'Towards communicative justice in health', *Medical Anthropology* 3 (4) (2017), 287–304.

Brown, Hannah, and Ann H. Kelly 'Material proximities and hotspots: Toward an anthropology of viral hemorrhagic fevers', *Medical Anthropology Quarterly* 28 (2) (2014), 280–303.

Cabalion, Sarah, Elmoubasher Abu Baker Abd Farag, Omer Abdelahdi, Hamad Al-Romaihi, and Frédéric Keck, 'Middle East respiratory syndrome coronavirus and human-camel relationships in Qatar', *Medicine Anthropology Theory* 5 (3) (2018), 177–194.

Caduff, Carlo 'On the verge of death: Visions of biological vulnerability', *Annual Review of Anthropology* 43 (2014), 105–121.

Caduff, Carlo *The Pandemic Perhaps: Dramatic Events in a Public Culture of Danger* (Berkeley, CA: The University of California Press, 2015).

Caprara, Andrea 'Cultural interpretations of contagion', *Tropical Medicine and International Health* 3 (12) (1998), 996–1001.

Chandler, Clare, Eleanor Hutchinson, and Coll Hutchison *Addressing Antimicrobial Resistance Through Social Theory: An Anthropologically Oriented Report* (London School of Hygiene & Tropical Medicine, 2016). www.lshtm.ac.uk/php/ghd/research/app/anthro pologyofantimicrobial resistance.html

Choy, Timothy K. 'Articulated knowledges: Environmental forms after universality's demise', *American Anthropologist* 107 (1) (2005), 5–18.

Cohn, Samuel K., Jr *Epidemics. Hate and Compassion from the Plague of Athens to AIDS* (Oxford: Oxford University Press, 2018).

Collier, Stephen J., Andrew Lakoff, and Paul Rabinow 'Biosecurity: Towards an anthropology of the contemporary', *Anthropology Today* 20 (5) (2004), 3–7.

Cooper, Melinda 'Pre-empting emergence: The biological turn in the war on terror', *Theory, Culture & Society* 23 (4) (2006), 113–135.

Craddock, Susan, and Steve Hinchliffee 'One world one health? Social science engagements with the one medicine agenda', *Social Science & Medicine* 129 (2015), 1–4.

Cunningham, Andrew 'Transforming plague: The laboratory and the identity of infectious disease', In Andrew Cunningham, and Perry Williams (eds.), *The Laboratory Revolution in Medicine*, pp. 209–244 (Cambridge: Cambridge University Press, 1992).

Danowski, Deborah, and Eduardo Viveiros de Castro *The Ends of the World*, translated by Rodrigo Nunes (Cambridge: Polity Press, 2016).

Das, Veena *Critical Events: An Anthropological Perspective on Contemporary India* (Oxford and New York: Oxford University Press, 1995).

Das, Veena, Arthur Kleinman, Margaret M. Lock, Mamphela Ramphele, and Pamela Reynolds, eds. *Remaking a World: Violence, Social Suffering, and Recovery* (Berkeley, CA: The University of California Press, 2001).

De Boeck, Filip. '"Divining" the city: Rhythm, amalgamation and knotting as forms of urbanity', *Social Dynamics* 41 (1) (2015), 47–58.

DeGroote, John P., Ramanathan Sugumaran, Sarah M. Brend, Brad J. Tucker, and Lyric C. Bartholomay 'Landscape, demographic, entomological, and climatic associations with human disease incidence of West Nile virus in the state of Iowa, USA', *International Journal of Health Geographics* 7 (19) (2008). https://doi.org/10.1186/1476-072X-7-19

DFID-Wellcome Trust DFID-Wellcome Joint Initiative on Epidemic Preparedness Call for Proposal (May 4, 2018). https://wellcome.ac.uk/sites/default/files/epidemic-prepared ness-social-science-research-protocols-call-for-proposals.pdf

Elbe, Stefan 'Risking lives: AIDS, security and three concepts of risk', *Security Dialogue* 39 (2–3) (2008), 177–198.

Engelmann, Lukas '"A source of sickness": Photographic mapping of the plague in Honolulu in 1900', In Lukas Engelmann, John Henderson, and Christos Lynteris (eds.), *Plague and the City*, pp. 139–158 (London and New York: Routledge, 2018).

Epelboin, Alain 'L'anthropologue dans la réponse aux épidémies: Science, savoir-faire ou placebo?' *Bulletin de l'AMADES. Anthropologie médicale appliquée au développement et à la santé* 78 (2009). https://journals.openedition.org/amades/1060

Erikson, Susan L. 'The financialization of Ebola', *Somatosphere* 11 (2015). http://somato sphere.net/2015/11/the-financialization-of-ebola.html

Esposito, Roberto *Immunitas: The Protection and Negation of Life* (London: Polity Press, 2011).

Evans, Nicholas H. A. 'Blaming the rat? Accounting for plague in colonial Indian medicine', *Medicine, Anthropology, Theory* 5 (3) (2018), 15–42.

Fairhead, James 'Postscript: Epidemic history and the Ebola present', In Christos Lynteris, and Nicholas H. A. Evans (eds.), *Histories of Post-Mortem Contagion: Infectious Corpses and Contested Burials*, pp. 113–121 (London: Palgrave Macmillan, 2018a).

Fairhead, James 'Technology, inclusivity and the rogue bats and the war against "the invisible enemy"', *Conservation and Society* 16 (2) Special Section: Green Wars (2018b), 170–180.

Farmer, Paul, et al. 'An anthropology of structural violence', *Current Anthropology* 45 (3) (2004), 305–325.

Farmer, Paul 'The second life of sickness: On structural violence and cultural humility', *Human Organization* 75 (4) (2016), 279–288.

Fassin, Didier *When Bodies Remember: Experiences and Politics of AIDS in South Africa* (Berkeley, CA: The University of California Press, 2007).

Feierman, Steven, and John Janzen, eds. *The Social Basis of Health and Healing in Africa* (Berkeley, CA: The University of California Press, 1992).

Fee, Elizabeth, and Theodore M. Brown 'Preemptive biopreparedness: Can we learn anything from history?' *American Journal of Public Health* 91 (5) (2001), 721–726.

Fontein, Joost 'Graves, ruins, and belonging: Towards an anthropology of proximity', *Journal of the Royal Anthropological Institute* 17 (2011), 706–727.

Fortané, Nicolas, and Frédéric Keck 'How biosecurity reframes animal surveillance', *Revue d'anthropologie des connaissances* 9 (2015), a–l. DOI:10.3917/rac.027.0126.URL

Fortun, Kim *Advocacy after Bhopal: Environmentalism, Disaster, New Global Orders* (Chicago, IL: The University of Chicago Press, 2009).

Fraustino, Julia Daisy and Liang Ma 'CDC'S use of social media and humor in a risk campaign – "Preparedness 101: Zombie Apocalypse"' *Journal of Applied Communication Research* 43 (2) (2015), 222–242.

Garrett, Laurie *The Coming Plague: Newly Emerging Diseases in a World out of Balance* (New York: Farrar, Straus, and Giroux, 1994).

Gomel, Elana 'The plague of utopias: Pestilence and the apocalyptic body', *Twentieth Century Literature* 46 (4) Literature and Apocalypse (2000), 405–433.

Grøn, Lone, and Lotte Meinert 'Social contagion and cultural epidemics: Phenomenological and "experience-near" explorations', *Ethnos* 45 (2) (2017), 165–181.

Halabi, Monique, Alexander Dao, Kyle Chen, and Brandon Brown 'Zombies – A pop culture resource for public health awareness', *Emerging Infectious Diseases* 19 (5) (2013), 809–813.

Hardon, Anita, and Hansjörg Dilger 'Global AIDS medicines in East African health institutions', *Medical Anthropology* 30 (2) (2011), 136–157.

Harrison, Mark *Contagion: How Commerce Has Spread Disease* (New Haven, CT: Yale University Press, 2012).

Harrison Mark 'Pandemics', In Mark Jackson (ed.), *The Routledge History of Disease* (London: Routledge, 2016).

Herring, D. Ann, and Alan C. Swedlund, eds. *Plagues and Epidemics: Infected Spaces Past and Present* (New York: Berg, 2010).

Hewlett, Bonnie S. and Barry L. Hewlett *Ebola, Culture and Politics: The Anthropology of an Emerging Disease* (Belmont, CA: Thomas Wadsworth Books, 2008).

Hinchliffe, Steve, and Kim J. Ward 'Geographies of folded life: How immunity reframes biosecurity', *Geoforum* 53 (2014), 136–144.

Hoppe, Kirk Arden *Lords of the Fly: Sleeping Sickness Control in British East Africa, 1900–1960* (Santa Barbara: Greenwood Publishing Group, 2003).

Inhorn, Marcia C., and Peter J. Brown 'The anthropology of infectious disease', *Annual Review of Anthropology* 19 (1) (1990), 89–117.

Janzen, John M. 'Afri-global medicine: New perspectives on epidemics, drugs, wars, migrations, and healing rituals', In Hansjörg Dilger, Abdoulaye Kane, and Stacey A. Langwick (eds.), *Medicine, Mobility, and Power in Global Africa: Transnational Health and Healing*, pp. 115–137 (Bloomington, IN: Indiana University Press, 2011).

Johnson, Pieter T. J., Alan R. Townsend, Cory C. Cleveland, Patricia M. Glibert, Robert W. Howarth, Valerie J. McKenzie, Eliska Rejmankova, and Mary H. Ward. 'Linking environmental nutrient enrichment and disease emergence in humans and wildlife', *Ecological Applications* 20 (1) (2010), 16–29.

Keck, Frédéric 'From mad cow disease to bird flu: Transformations of food safety in France', In Andrew Lakoff, and Stephen J. Collier (eds.), *Biosecurity Interventions: Global Health and Security in Question*, pp. 195–227 (New York: Columbia University Press, 2008).

Keck, Frédéric 'Ebola, entre science et fiction', *Anthropologie & Santé* 11 (2015). http://jour nals.openedition.org/anthropologiesante/1870. DOI: 10.4000/anthropologiesante.1870

Keck, Frédéric, and Christos Lynteris 'Zoonosis: prospects and challenges for medical anthropology', *Medicine Anthropology Theory* 5 (3) (2018), 1–14. https://doi.org/ 10. 17157/mat.5.3.372.

Keck, Frédéric, and Andrew Lakoff 'Sentinel devices', *Limn* 3 (2015). https://limn.it/ articles/preface-sentinel-devices-2/

Kelly, Ann H. 'Ebola vaccines, evidentiary charisma and the rise of global health emergency research', *Economy and Society* 47 (1) (2018), 135–161.

Kelly, Ann H., and Javier Lezaun 'The wild indoors: Room-spaces of scientific inquiry', *Cultural Anthropology* 32 (3) (2017), 367–398.

Kelly, Ann H., and Almudena Marí-Sáez 'Shadowlands and dark corners: Towards an anthropology of light and zoonosis', *Medicine Anthropology Theory* 5 (3) (2018). DOI: 10.17157/mat.5.3.382

Kienzler, Hanna 'Debating war-trauma and post-traumatic stress disorder (PTSD) in an interdisciplinary arena', *Social Science & Medicine* 67 (2) (2008), 218–227.

King, Nicholas B. 'Security, disease, commerce: Ideologies of postcolonial global health', *Social Studies of Science* 32 (5–6) *Postcolonial Technoscience* (October–December 2002), 763–789.

King, Nicholas B. 'The scale politics of emerging diseases', *Osiris* 2nd Series 19 Landscapes of Exposure: Knowledge and Illness in Modern Environments (2004), 62–76.

Kleinman, Arthur 'Local worlds of suffering: An interpersonal focus for ethnographies of illness experience', *Qualitative Health Research* 2 (2) (1992), 127–134.

Kosoy, Michael 'Deepening the conception of functional information in the description of zoonotic infectious diseases', *Entropy* 15 (5) (2013), 1929–1962.

Kruvand, Marjorie and Maggie Silver 'Zombies gone viral: How a fictional invasion helped CDC promote emergency preparedness', *Case Studies in Strategic Communication* 2 (2013), 34–60.

Lachenal, Guillaume 'Ebola 2014: Chronicle of a well-prepared disaster' *Somatosphere* (October 31, 2014). http://somatosphere.net/2014/10/chronicle-of-a-well-prepared-dis aster.html

Lachenal, Guillaume 'Lessons in medical nihilism: Virus hunters, neoliberalism and the AIDS crisis in Cameroon', In P. Wenzel Geissler (ed.), *Para-States and Medical Science: Making African Global Health*, pp. 103–41 (Durham, NC: Duke University Press, 2015).

Lainé, Nicolas 'Elephant tuberculosis as a reverse zoonosis. Postcolonial scenes of compassion, conservation, and public health in Laos and France', *Medicine Anthropology Theory* 5 (3) (2018), 157–176.

Lakoff, Andrew 'Two regimes of global health', *Humanity: An International Journal of Human Rights, Humanitarianism, and Development* 1 (1) (2010), 59–79.

Landecker, Hannah 'Antibiotic resistance and the biology of history', *Body and Society* 22 (4) (2016), 19–52.

Latour, Bruno *The Pasteurization of France*, translated by Alan Sheridan (Cambridge, MA: Harvard University Press, 1993).

Leach, Melissa, and Ian Scoones 'The social and political lives of zoonotic disease models: Narratives, science and policy', *Social Science & Medicine* 88 (2013), 10–17.

Leach, Melissa, and Mariz Tadros 'Epidemics and the politics of knowledge: Contested narratives in Egypt's H1N1 response', *Medical Anthropology* 33 (3) (2014), 240–254.

Wilkinson, Annie, and Melissa Leach 'Briefing: Ebola–myths, realities, and structural violence', *African Affairs* 114 (454) (2015), 136–148.

Lezaun, Javier, and Catherine M. Montgomery 'The pharmaceutical commons: Sharing and exclusion in global health drug development', *Science, Technology, & Human Values* 40 (1) (2015), 3–29.

Lindenbaum Shirley *Kuru Sorcery: Disease and Danger in the New Guinea Highlands* (Palo Alto, CA: Mayfield, 1979).

Lindenbaum, Shirley 'Kuru, prions, and human affairs: Thinking about epidemics', *Annual Review of Anthropology* 30 (1) (2001), 363–385.

Lock, Margaret, and Vinh-Kim Nguyen *An Anthropology of Biomedicine* (New York: Wiley-Blackwell, 2010).

Lockrem, Jessica, and Adonia Lugo 'Infrastructures' *Cultural Anthropology Blog* (2015). https://culanth.org/curated_collections/11-infrastructure

Lowe, Celia 'Viral ethnography: Metaphors for writing life', *RCC Perspectives* (1) (2017), 91–96. Doi.org/10.5282/rcc/7779.

Löwy, Ilana 'Making plagues visible', In D. Ann Herring, and Alan C. Swedlund (eds.), *Plagues and Epidemics: Infected Spaces Past and Present*, pp. 269–286 (New York: Berg, 2010).

Lloyd-Smith, James O., Sebastian J. Schreiber, P. Ekkehard Kopp, and Wayne M. Getz 'Superspreading and the effect of individual variation on disease emergence', *Nature* 438 (7066) (2005), 355–359.

Lynteris, Christos 'Epidemics as events and as crises: Comparing two plague outbreaks in Manchuria (1910–11 and 1920–21)', *The Cambridge Journal of Anthropology* 32 (1) (Spring 2014), 62–76.

Lynteris, Christos *Ethnographic Plague: Configuring Disease on the Chinese-Russian Frontier* (London: Palgrave Macmillan, 2016a).

Lynteris, Christos 'The prophetic faculty of epidemic photography: Chinese wet markets and the imagination of the next pandemic', *Visual Anthropology* 29 (2) Medicine, Photography and Anthropology (2016b), 118–132.

Lynteris, Christos 'The epidemiologist as culture hero: Visualizing humanity in the age of "the next pandemic"', *Visual Anthropology* 29 (1) (January 2016c), 36–53.

Lynteris, Christos 'A suitable soil: Plague's breeding grounds at the dawn of the third pandemic', *Medical History* 61 (3) (June 2017a), 343–357.

Lynteris, Christos 'Zoonotic diagrams: Mastering and unsettling human-animal relations', *Journal of the Royal Anthropological Institute* N.S. 23 (3) (September 2017b), 463–485.

Lynteris, Christos 'Pestis minor: The history of a contested plague pathology', *Bulletin of the History of Medicine* (in print).

Lynteris, Christos, and Nicholas H. A. Evans 'Introduction: The challenge of the epidemic corpse', In Christos Lynteris, and Nicholas H. A. Evans (eds.), *Histories of Post-Mortem Contagion: Infectious Corpses and Contested Burials*, pp. 1–26 (London: Palgrave Macmillan, 2018).

Magnusson, Bruce, and Zahi A. Zalloua 'Introduction: The Hydra of contagion', In Bruce Magnusson, and Zahi A. Zalloua (eds.), *Contagion: Health, Fear Sovereignty*, pp. 3–24 (Seattle: University of Washington Press, 2012).

Malinowski, Bronislaw 'Practical anthropology', *Africa* 2 (1) (1929), 22–38.

Martineau, Fred, Annie Wilkinson, and Melissa Parker 'Epistemologies of Ebola: Reflections on the experience of the Ebola response anthropology platform', *Anthropological Quarterly* 90 (2) (2017), 475–494.

Masco, Joseph *The Theater of Operations: National Security Affect from the Cold War to the War on Terror* (Durham, NC: Duke University Press, 2014).

Massumi, Brian *Ontopower: War, Powers, and the State of Perception* (Durham, NC: Duke University Press, 2015).

Mendelsohn, J. Andrew ' "Like all that lives": Biology, medicine and bacteria in the age of Pasteur and Koch', *History and Philosophy of the Life Sciences* 24 (1) (2002), 3–36.

Mitropoulos, Angela *Contract & Contagion: From Biopolitics to Oikonomia* (New York: Minor Compositions, 2012).

Nading, Alex M. 'Local biologies, leaky things, and the chemical infrastructure of global health', *Medical Anthropology* 36 (2) (2017), 141–156.

Neill, Deborah *Networks in Tropical Medicine: Internationalism, Colonialism, and the Rise of a Medical Specialty, 1890–1930* (Stanford, CA: Stanford University Press, 2012).

Nichter, Mark, and Mimi Nichter *Anthropology and International Health* (London and New York: Routledge, 1996).

Nuñes, João 'Ebola and the production of neglect in global health', *Third World Quarterly* 37 (3) (2016), 542–556.

Ostherr, Kirsten *Cinematic Prophylaxis: Globalization and Contagion in the Discourse of World Health* (Durham, NC: Duke University Press, 2005).

Peckham, Robert 'Economies of contagion: Financial crisis and pandemic', *Economy and Society* 42 (2) (2013), 226–248.

Pigg, Stacy Leigh 'Found in most traditional societies. Traditional medical practitioners between culture and development', In Cooper, Frederick, and Randall M. Packard (eds.), *International Development and the Social Sciences, Essays on the History and Politics of Knowledge*, pp. 259–290 (Berkeley, CA: The University of California Press, 1997).

Poleykett, Branwyn 'Pasteurian tropical medicine and colonial scientific vision', *Subjectivity* 10 (2) (2017), 190–203.

Poleykett, Branwyn 'Ethnohistory and the dead: Cultures of colonial epidemiology', *Medical Anthropology* (2018). DOI:10.1080/01459740.2018.1453507

Porter, Natalie 'Bird flu biopower: Strategies for multispecies coexistence in Việt Nam', *American Ethnologist* 40 (1) (2013), 132–148.

Preston, Richard *The Hot Zone* (New York: Random House, 1994).

Quammen, David *Spillover: Animal Infections and the Next Human Pandemic* (New York: W. W. Norton & Company, 2012).

Richards, Paul *Ebola: How a People's Science Helped to End an Epidemic* (London: Zed Books, 2016).

Robbins, Steve 'The colour of science', *Journal of Southern African Studies* 30 (3) (2004), 651–672.

Rosenberg, Charles E. *Explaining Epidemics* (Cambridge: Cambridge University Press, 1992).

Rosental, Paul A. 'Où s'arrête la contagion? Faits et utopie chez Gabriel Tarde', *Tracés. Revue de sciences humaines* 21 (2) (2011), 109–124.

Sampson, Tony D. *Virality: Contagion Theory in the Age of Networks* (Minneapolis: Minnesota University Press, 2012).

Sams, Kelley, Alice Desclaux, Julienne Anoko, Francis Akindès, Marc Egrot, Khoudia Sow, Bernard Taverne, et al. 'Mobilising experience from Ebola to address plague in Madagascar and future epidemics', *The Lancet* 390 (10113) (2017), 2624–2625.

Scheper-Hughes, Nancy, and Margaret M. Lock 'Speaking 'truth' to illness: Metaphors, reification, and a pedagogy for patients', *Medical Anthropology Quarterly* 17 (5) (1986), 137–140.

Schoepf, Brooke G. 'International AIDS research in anthropology: Taking a critical perspective on the crisis', *Annual Review of Anthropology* 30 (1) (2001), 335–361.

Schumaker, Lyn *Africanizing Anthropology: Fieldwork, Networks and the Making of Cultural Knowledge in Central Africa* (Durham, NC: Duke University Press, 2001).

Servitje, Lorenzo, and Megan Nixon 'The making of a modern endemic: An introduction', In Megan Nixon, and Lorenzo Servitje (eds.), *Endemic: Essays in Contagion Theory*, pp. 1–17 (London: Palgrave Macmillan, 2016).

Silver, Maggie *Preparedness 101: Zombie Pandemic* (Atlanta: Centers for Disease Control, U.S. Department of Health and Human Services, 2011).

Simone, AbdouMaliq 'People as infrastructure: Intersecting fragments in Johannesburg', *Public Culture* 16 (3) (2004), 407–429.

Singer, Merrill 'The spread of Zika and the potential for global arbovirus syndemics', *Global Public Health* 12 (1) (2017), 1–18.

Smith, Shawn Michelle *At the Edge of Sight: Photography and the Unseen* (Durham, NC: Duke University Press, 2013).

Stellmach, Derryl 'Research protocol: The practice of medical humanitarian emergency: Ethnography of practitioners', *Response to nutritional crisis* (Oxford, UK, 2013). http://hdl.handle.net/10144/323862

Stellmach, Derryl, Isabelle Beshar, Juliette Bedford, Philipp du Cors, and Beverley Stringer 'Anthropology in public health emergencies: What is anthropology good for?' *British Medical Journal Global Health* 3 (2) (2018), e000534. DOI:10.1136/bmjgh-2017-000534

Sunder Rajan, Kaushik *Biocapital: The Constitution of Postgenomic Life* (Durham, NC: Duke University Press, 2006).

Schweitzer, Dahlia *Going Viral: Zombies, Viruses, and the End of the World* (New Brunswick: Rutgers University Press, 2018).

Tilley, Helen *Africa as a Living Laboratory: Empire, Development, and the Problem of Scientific Knowledge, 1870–1950* (Chicago, IL: The University of Chicago Press, 2011).

Trostle, James 'Anthropology and epidemiology in the twentieth century: A selective history of collaborative projects and theoretical affinities, 1920 to 1970', In Craig R. Janes, Ron Stall, and Sandra M. Gifford (eds.), *Anthropology and Epidemiology: Interdisciplinary Approaches to the Study of Health and Disease*, pp. 59–94 (Dordrecht: D. Reidel Publishing Company, 1986).

Tsing, Anna *Friction: An Ethnography of Global Connection* (Princeton, NJ: Princeton University Press, 2004).

Vaughan, Megan *Curing their Ills: Colonial Power and African Illness* (Stanford, CA: Stanford University Press, 1991).

Wald, Priscilla *Contagious: Cultures, Carriers, and the Outbreak Narrative* (Durham, NC: Duke University Press, 2008).

Wilkinson, Annie, and Melissa Leach 'Briefing: Ebola – myths, realities, and structural violence', *African Affairs* 114 (454) (2015), 136–148.

Wolf, Meike, and Kevin Hall. 'Cyborg preparedness: Incorporating knowing and caring bodies into emergency infrastructures', *Medical Anthropology* (2018), 1–13. DOI:10.10 80/01459740.2018.1485022

Wolfe, Nathan *The Viral Storm: The Dawn of a New Pandemic Age* (New York: Penguin Books, 2011).

World Health Organisation [WHO] 'Report of the Ebola interim assessment panel' (2015). www.who.int/csr/resources/publications/ebola/ebola-panel-report/en/

World Health Organisation [WHO] 'Integrating social science interventions in epidemic, pandemic and health emergencies response: Report of the informal consultation' (June 8, 2017). http://apps.who.int/iris/bitstream/handle/10665/259933/WHO-WHE-IHM-2018.1-eng.pdf?sequence=1

1 Simulations of epidemics

Techniques of global health and neo-liberal government

Frédéric Keck and Guillaume Lachenal

In the last twenty years, techniques of simulation have multiplied in the world of disaster management. They have been applied to all hazards of collective life: earthquakes, floods, terrorist attacks, climate change, as well as new infectious diseases. These different types of events, despite the obvious contrasts between natural and intentional, short-term and long-term, have in common their low probability and catastrophic consequences, opening a temporality of emergency and calling for quick action. Simulation is used when virtual threats cannot be calculated as risks but must be anticipated as if they had already actualised. It is a technique of imagination to immerge in the reality of future disasters and mitigate their catastrophic effects.

How has public health been transformed by the treatment of emerging infectious diseases through simulation? How has the use of fiction and scenarios changed the management of public health? How has it transformed the concept of epidemics by managing infectious diseases not in a territory that could be controlled and contained through quarantine and vaccination, but in a global space where they could emerge at any point and should be monitored and anticipated on all points?

If simulations of future epidemics rely on scenarios of past epidemics based on the memories of public health actors, they also involve fiction on a larger scale: that of a planet connected by networks of surveillance where every outbreak of a new infectious disease is detected through early warning signals and mitigated before a pandemic occurs. This fiction – based on the memory of past pandemics among global health experts – has gaps and flaws: it leaves aside neglected diseases, wrong signals, lured sentinels. This chapter will explore these disjunctions in the world of epidemic simulation by looking at the behaviour of actors when they have to stage a simulation in local contexts.

Gaps and flaws in the simulation of epidemics have been described by anthropologists in North America where these techniques have first been implemented in the context of the end of the Cold War as a result of the transfer of techniques of anticipation from nuclear deterrence to all-hazards management (Caduff 2015; Lakoff 2017). These researchers have showed that the shift in rationalities of risk from prevention to preparedness has opened a vacuum space in which actors can formulate criticisms of public health, often in terms of the precautionary principle. Why, actors ask, should we prepare for an epidemic that will not be the same

DOI: 10.4324/9780429461897-2

as past epidemics, given the mutability of pathogens and the variability of their conditions of emergence?

Our chapter proposes to move beyond the transatlantic Euro-American province (Chakrabarty 2000), which has remained the reference point of most works on pandemics (e.g. Zylberman 2013), drawing from our ethnographic work in Africa and Asia. The criticisms we have observed in stages of epidemic simulation in these contexts don't rely on the same arguments. Rather, they question the distraction of resources that simulation exercises represent, as they mobilise finances, staff, vehicles, and spaces in context of generalised scarcity, by framing simulation exercises as a ritual of compliance to global standards and donor priorities. They invoke the lack of realism of the simulation to turn fiction against itself, playing on the different modes of engagement in the planned scenario (Revet 2013). The criticism of the reality of the extraordinary epidemics to which simulation should prepare, opposed to the reality of ordinary public health, thus opens margins of distanciation within the stage of the simulation. Beyond the mediatic images of simulations produced by public health authorities, actors themselves, often coming from lower ranks of health services, express irony or critique to distance themselves from the scenario. Drawing from the anthropology of ritual, we will analyse what simulation does to the competences of the actors involved, and how they manage to perform the simulation without believing in the reality of the epidemic to come.

We will thus combine a history of public health and an anthropology of rituals to examine the margins of simulation, both in the sense of the margins of global health and the margins of the exercise. Rather than describe simulation from the centre of public health planners in North America, we will analyse how they are staged and criticised by actors who are involved in it from the margins of the global community. Because we believe that simulations of epidemics will proliferate as techniques of neo-liberal government in the years to come, we want to open fields for research in ethnography and history of global health.

Scenarios as anticipations of the past

Since scenarios are techniques for mitigating the uncertainty of the future by preparing for catastrophic events as if these had already occurred (Sunstein 2007), they may appear, at first sight, as products of the imagination. The use of scenarios to anticipate future disasters is often attributed to Herman Kahn, an American expert in futurology who joined the RAND Corporation after the Second World War to advise the US government on how to wage a thermonuclear war (Zylberman 2013: 28, 153; Hamblin 2013: 153–155; Galison 2014; Lakoff 2017: 23–24). Kahn is famous among futurologists for orienting game theory as a mathematical technique toward 'thinking the unthinkable'; that is, introducing in mathematical models the possibility of life after a nuclear bomb. Kahn used scenarios as ways to introduce 'the unthinkable' into a reasonable series of events. He wrote:

> A scenario results from an attempt to describe in more or less detail some hypothetical sequence of events. The scenario is particularly suited to dealing

with several aspects of a problem more or less simultaneously, [helping us] get a feel for events and the branching points dependent upon critical choices.

(Kahn 1962: 143)

In his view, scenarios aimed at immerging decision makers in a world transformed by the disaster to stimulate their imagination. 'Imagination', he argued, 'has always been one of the principal means for dealing in various ways with the future, and the scenario is simply one of the many devices useful in stimulating and disciplining the imagination' (Kahn 1962: 145). In the games he designed for the RAND Corporation players were divided into opposing teams representing states at war, and the game director played secondary actors as well as 'nature', whose function was to introduce chance events into the game (Ghamari-Tabrizi 2005: 151).

> Participants were reluctant to use the word "game" to describe these exercises (preferring "simulation"), since game seemed an unsuitable name for rehearsals of conventional, limited, or all-out nuclear war. The phrase "serious play" characterised war-gaming in the heaps of articles introducing it to military audiences.
>
> (Ibid.: 160)

Kahn's ideas about imagination of the unthinkable and the RAND's game theory were borrowed by the applied mathematician Robert Kupperman who worked at the Office of Emergency Preparedness (OEP) in the early 1970s and later in the Center for Strategic and International Studies (CSIS). Kupperman emphasised the role of simulation exercises in training for crisis management: 'Ideally', he wrote, 'when a real crisis hits, no difference should exist, either operationally or emotionally, between the current reality and the previous training simulations' (Kupperman 1983: 202, quoted in Lakoff 2017: 48). In the 1990s, this technique was used by experts in microbiology and epidemiology to convince national security experts they needed to prepare for attacks using bioweapons. Donald Henderson, who had directed the World Health Organization's successful smallpox eradication programme, argued with Richard Clarke, counter-terrorism adviser under Presidents George H.W. Bush and Bill Clinton, that the US population was not immune to an attack of smallpox which could be launched from anywhere, as revealed by the Soviet defector Ken Alibek (Lakoff 2017: 50). Nobel-prize winning microbiologist Joshua Lederberg explained the emergence of new viruses such as Ebola in 1976 by the changing relations between humans and their environment (deforestation, urbanisation, industrialisation of agriculture and animal husbandry, mass transportation). Despite the success of the vaccination campaign against major infectious diseases such as smallpox, declared eradicated in 1980, he claimed, 'we have never been so vulnerable', encouraging public health experts to anticipate pathogens in decentralised networks of information rather than protect populations in national territories (King 2002, 2004). Simulations of epidemics were then used by public health experts and national security advisers as techniques to imagine and assess the vulnerabilities of social life's infrastructures (Collier and Lakoff 2015).

On June 22–23, 2001, the Johns Hopkins Center for Civilian Biodefense created three years before by Donald Henderson, in collaboration with the CSIS and the ANSER Institute for Homeland Security, organised an exercise called 'Dark Winter', which simulated a large-scale smallpox attack from Iraq on the United States. The organisers recruited twelve prominent public figures to serve as role players, as well as an audience of more than a hundred observers. The exercise took place in three segments over two days, depicting a time-span of two weeks after the initial biological attack. The controllers of the exercise introduced information on the depletion of vaccine stocks and the growing panics over remaining doses, which led the decision makers to discuss whether they would use the National Guard to enforce quarantine. The Director of CSIS, John Hamre, narrated the final stage of the exercise:

> In the last 48 hours, there were 14,000 cases. We now have 1,000 dead, another 5,000 that we expect to be dead within weeks. There are 200 people who died from the vaccination, because there is a small percentage [of risk], and we have administered 12 million doses. . . . At this stage, the medical system is completely overwhelmed.
>
> (quoted in Lakoff 2017: 55)

Most actors and observers esteemed with astonishment that the exercise revealed the lack of preparedness in the US for a bioweapon attack – just a few months before the anthrax letters following the 9/11 attacks increased this feeling. Richard Clarke had organised such exercises with government officials secretly ('Blair House' in March 1998, simulating an Ebola outbreak in the US, based on the novel of Richard Preston (1998), *The Cobra Event*) and similar simulations were set up in Washington with international actors and observers in the following years ('Atlantic Storm' in January 2005, simulating a smallpox attack from Al-Qaida in Europe and the US). But no exercise had a similar effect on public health investments as 'Dark Winter'. Note that all these simulations took place on computers in an office in Washington DC.

Beyond these landmark examples, scenario-making in public health simulations requires much more than imagination – be it nurtured by trauma, science fiction, or fantasy. Epidemic scenarios specifically mobilise a politics and a practice of remembering, involving references to popular memory as well as historical research and systematic 'digging' into public health records. They also draw their authority from the ever-improving science of *in-silico* epidemic modelling, which has recently benefited from the progress of phylogenetic studies (aiming at the reconstitution of the history of pathogen spread based on their genetic sequences through computer work, by contrast with *in vivo* and in *vitro* biological research). For instance, the scenario of a smallpox attack in the US was not based on scientific precedents, but rather on the traumatic memory of the effects of smallpox on the American continent in the past centuries, where it intentionally and unintentionally killed millions of Native Americans (Diamond 1997; Wolfe et al. 2007). The Dark Winter exercise was also based on historical data on the transmission patterns of actual past smallpox outbreaks between 1958 and 1973 to assume the rate of disease transmission that gave its tempo to the exercise. The generalisation of simulation exercises as part of global health security programmes following the SARS and avian flu crises in 2003–05 (see the following) co-produced a renewed interest for the history of influenza pandemics and especially for the 1918 pandemic (Giles-Vernick and Craddock 2010). The reference to the 'Spanish flu' pandemic as the historical precedent that can help think the unthinkable has become commonplace in the global health community – the perfect 'wake-up call' and a classic preamble in simulation exercises (Zylberman 2013: 21). As a recent example, intervening in major global media during the carefully orchestrated launching of the Coalition for Pandemic Preparedness Innovation (CEPI) in 2015 (Yong 2018) announced repeatedly that, according to modellers, '33 million people could die in 250 days' if a severe flu pandemic occurred – the (unsourced) figure went viral in most press releases on the CEPI creation.

Influenza is estimated to have killed from twenty to fifty million persons between 1918 and 1920 – more than the war itself. While the epidemiological analysis is difficult to establish because of war censorship (hence the name 'Spanish flu': Spain, being a neutral country, reported all its cases, including the king himself), the first cases were reported in Haskell County, Kansas, in January 1918; then in Europe, Africa, and Asia with a lethality rate of around ten percent. The next pandemic influenza virus was identified in 1957 in Singapore and caused two million casualties as it moved from East to West and another one in was identified in Hong Kong in 1968 causing one million casualties. After the Second World War, influenza viruses were classified by their hemaglutinin and neuraminidase proteins commanding the entrance and release of the virus into the cell: H1N1 in 1918, H2N2 in 1957, H3N2 in 1968. The role of birds as reservoir of the disease being established in the 1960s by Australian scientists; influenza viruses in birds were monitored to anticipate the next pandemic virus (Shortridge and Stuart-Harris 1982). Hence the alert raised in Hong Kong in 1997 when the H5N1 virus killed five thousand chickens (with almost twenty percent of Hong Kong chickens infected) and eight persons out of the twelve who contracted the disease and then spread from China to Europe and Africa (Smith et al. 2006). The scenario of a flu virus emerging from Chinese birds and transmitted through the hubs of Hong Kong and Singapore to the rest of the world became credible in the 1990s with the development of the Chinese economy and the fears of the consequences of the return of Hong Kong and Macao under Chinese sovereignty (MacPhail 2014; Mason 2016). Debates have raged in the last twenty years whether the 1918 epidemic started in the US or in China (Hanoun 1993; Taubenberger 2006; Humphries 2014). It has also been estimated based on phylogenic reconstruction that the H1N1 virus was circulating among pigs as early as 1911 before emerging among humans as a pandemic in 1918 and then becoming seasonal (Smith et al. 2009).

HIV/AIDS has similarly seen historical epidemiology being used as a cautionary tale. In this case phylogenetic studies and historical research have enabled the reconstruction of a consensus scenario explaining the appearance and spread of HIV among human populations in the twentieth century (Giles-Vernick 2013), making it the ultimate example of a zoonotic emergence that went wrong – an event of zoonotic transmission from chimpanzees to humans leading to a forty-million deaths pandemic in less than a century as a result of a 'perfect storm' (Pépin 2011) of biological bad luck, of social and ecological change associated with colonial rule, of hazardous technological interventions (blood transfusions and injections), and of political inaction when the epidemic was eventually detected in the 1980s. Influenza pandemics and the HIV/AIDS pandemic are thus paradigmatic examples of how 'lessons of history' generate political awareness of unpreparedness and in turn can help calibrate epidemic models and scenarios for exercises and contingency plans.

The case of the Ebola virus suggests a less straightforward link between histori-cal memory, simulations, and preparedness. The 1976 Ebola outbreak has deeply marked international health, and its memory has been instrumental in the forma-tion of the 'Emerging Infectious Diseases' worldview (King 2002) – the 1976 team airlifted to Yambuku in Zaire involved future prominent global health specialists such as Peter Piot and Joseph McCormick. Yet, according to most observers, the fiasco of the response to the epidemic of 2014–15 in West Africa was due not to lack of memory but to the fact that an epidemic of this scale and in that region was not considered to be in the realm of the possible, based on historical experi-ence (almost all epidemics had occurred in Central Africa, and never reached such proportions); it was also pointed that the much criticised 'over-reaction' of the WHO to the H1N1 epidemic in 2009 led to a systematic underplay of the new crisis. In other words, it was the very presence of the past as a source of anticipa-tion (and not its forgetting) that enabled the inaction of most global health actors. The West African epidemic had not appeared in a void space (Lachenal 2014) but in a zone (Eastern Sierra Leone) with a long history of US-funded programmes of hemmorragic fevers surveillance (notably in Kenema) and occurred after a decade of implementation of preparedness policies in African countries under the guid-ance of international organisations such as the OCHA, the FAO, and the CDC. The very status of Ebola as a top-of-the-agenda emerging threat – in the domain of exception, military research, and fiction – seems to have actually 'unprepared' African countries and international health organisations: they seemed literally unable to process what was happening in 2014 in the outbreak zone, for the fram-ing of Ebola as a fascinating 'jungle virus' rendered it unbelievable, which led to weeks of paralysis and even active denial of the seriousness of the epidemic by the WHO in the crucial months of May–July 2014 (MSF 2015). Given the result-ing debacle, it may be said that, by making the actual epidemic unthinkable, the apocalyptic fictions about Ebola (such as Richard Preston's 1994 and 1998 best sellers) had taken a performative, or even prophetic, dimension.

The 2014–15 Ebola fiasco also notoriously concerned computer simula-tions of the epidemics, with models alternatively predicting quick extinction or . . . holocaust – the most famous simulation produced by CDC modellers in

September 2014 announced 1.4 million deaths in Liberia by Christmas (Brown 2015). But beyond that spectacular over-estimation (which had the merit of mobilising donors and governments) the modelling of epidemics has considerably improved, and enables precise, parametric, calibrations of scenarios of epidemics and of their consequences (from the number of casualties to the economic effects on the national gross product). In addition to elaborated models of transmission, the use (and real-time sharing among the scientific community) of genetic sequences, allowing the building of phylogenetic trees and the retro-calculation of the epidemic history (through methods based on Bayesian coalescence theory) now enable real-time following and analysis of epidemics – as was demonstrated during the Zika epidemic (Faria et al. 2017). Phylogenetic studies, by definition, use traces of the past (genetic sequences, which are ever-actualised recapitulations of evolutionary history) as a way to understand ongoing epidemic processes and to forecast the near and distant futures.

How far is this use of the past to anticipate the future specific to epidemics? The role of scenarios in warning for future environmental threats has been stressed in different domains of science studies. Epidemic scenarios hold an intermediary position between scenarios of terrorist attacks and scenarios of climate change. For terrorist attacks, simulations rely on past scenarios to explore imagined possibilities in a virtual space of the imagination (Samimian-Darash 2016). For climate change, simulations rely on models that take a linear form with tipping points, to adapt to future changes in the environment (Sismondo 1999). For infectious diseases, simulations rely on models based on bioinformatics, displaying the beginning and end of the curve, anticipating different waves of the epidemic (Mackenzie 2003). Modellers act as poker players asking what would have happened if they had behaved differently given a mutation of the pathogen. Natasha Schull proposes the term 'reverse scenarios' in her work with online gamblers, to describe the way they 'cope with the necessarily uncertain futures of any hand by returning them to a point in the past and confronting them with a branching diversity of outcomes that might have emerged from it' (Schull 2015: 56). Anticipation is thus a way to inscribe the future in the past by rewriting the past through scenarios of future threats.

> Anticipation is not just betting on the future; it is a moral economy in which the future sets the conditions of possibility for action in the present, in which the future is inhabited in the present. Through anticipation, the future arrives as already formed in the present, as if the emergency has already happened.
>
> (Adams et al. 2009: 249)

In the next section, we will see how 'reverse scenarios' of infectious diseases work in practice, after describing in this first section their emergence as techniques for the imaginary management of future threats. We will also show how they have spread from the US to the rest of the world as techniques of anticipation of future epidemics and been transformed in their local contexts of implementation.

Standardisation through exercises

The success of 'Dark Winter' in 2001 in demonstrating the potential failures of US preparedness led to a blossoming of such exercises in public health institutions in the following years:

> In the United States, hospitals are required to stage at least one exercise per year with a simulated patient suffering from a highly communicable disease. The aim of such testing through exercises and drills is to assess pandemic preparedness; that is, to evaluate performance, ensure compliance, maintain vigilance, and improve readiness. Simulated events allow public health professionals to reveal potential vulnerabilities and address gaps in the preparedness and response plans. Tabletop exercises result in after-action reports and improvement plans, where procedures are reviewed and recommendations made.
>
> (Caduff 2015: 130)

At the national level, the 'Top Officials' series of terrorism preparedness exercises began with a simulated biological attack in 2000 and TOPOFF scenarios are staged every other year in multiple sites. For instance, TOPOFF 4, held in 2007, involved more than 15,000 participants from three international governments and included citizen participants role-playing victims and local emergency responders reacting in real time as the event unfolded (Armstrong 2012: 109).

The European Commission in Brussels also organised epidemic scenarios after 2002 and the planning of these simulations was one of the tasks of the European Center for Disease Controls created in 2004 and based in Stockholm (Zylberman 2013: 310). In Europe, however, scenarios of public health crises have mostly started with a food safety problem, such as a contamination of the food chain by bacteria, rather than by a terrorist attack. In 2003, the emergence of SARS in China, which caused thirty-two cases of infection in Europe but no deaths (although it killed ten percent of the 8,000 persons it infected globally), confirmed experts' scenarios on the emergence of new infectious diseases from the animal reservoir in south China. European scenarios of epidemics increasingly came to start with a SARS-like virus.

In the Asia-Pacific, exercises of simulation have been organised by public health authorities after the SARS outbreak, considered as the first pandemic of the twentieth century and putting Asia at the centre stage of global health (Abraham 2007). On June 7–8, 2006, Singapore and Australia organised a desktop exercise for the twenty-one members of the Asia-Pacific Economic Cooperation. The Exercise Coordination Centre was based in Canberra, from where information was sent to the twenty-one members of the public health staff about how the scenario would unfold. An outbreak of human-to-human H5N1 influenza was reported in Singapore (called 'Straits Flu'); the WHO had upgraded the alert from phase 4 to phase 5; a warehouse that manufactures personal protection equipment had burned; teams were flying to Vietnam for an APEC football tournament;

backpackers and fishermen started to get sick around the area of the outbreak. . . . On August 14–15, Singapore hosted a post-exercise workshop in which participants agreed that, 'The exercise provided an excellent opportunity to establish and test a communication network and to develop relationships between the economies' (UNSIC 2008, 63).

Similarly, on November 13, 2006, Hong Kong coordinated a desktop exercise called 'Great Wall' in which the health departments of Hong Kong, Macau, Jiangsu, and Beijing had to manage a virtual cluster of three human infections with H5N1 in a family after their visit to a poultry market. As one of the members of the family was supposed to travel from Jiangsu to Hong Kong and Macau, the goal of the exercise was 'to synchronize the three systems (of pandemic response) to engender an effective response among them' (UNSIC 2008: 18). The exercise opened with a ceremony attended by the Vice-Minister of the Chinese Ministry of Health, Wang Longde. It was considered as a success in creating good relations between mainland China and the former British and Portuguese colonies.

In Hong Kong, the Centre for Health Protection, created by the Department of Health after the SARS crisis to anticipate similar outbreaks through active surveillance and communication, is in charge through its Emergency Response Branch to write scenarios of epidemics and organise simulations not only indoors, such as Great Wall, but also outdoors in live poultry markets, slaughterhouses, airports, residential buildings, and hospitals. Occuring twice a year, these field exercises have borne names of natural phenomena – Maple, Cypress, Chestnut, Redwood, Eagle, Mountain Hua – as if to show that diseases were part of the natural ecosystem of the territory. There was no other epidemic simulation in Hong Kong in 2009, because the Emergency Response Branch considered the management of the H1N1 virus in the spring and autumn to be a 'real-life exercise'.

In January 2009, 'Exercise Redwood' took place in the clinic of Shau Kei Wan, located in the working-class district of Hong Kong island. The following scenario was distributed to the participants and posted at major public buildings. Confirmed cases of avian influenza with human infection had been reported in Hong Kong's neighbouring countries, as well as a rising trend in patient attendance with influenza-like illness in Hong Kong hospitals. Live poultry tested positive for influenza in Hong Kong's markets and were then culled at farms and markets. A member of the staff participating in the culling was reported to have the H5N1 virus, as well as an eight-year-old boy who had played with live poultry. Four clinics were designated in Hong Kong to triage patients with influenza-like illness and send patients with H5N1 to emergency departments. Only the final part of the scenario was performed in Shau Kei Wan; the first part was meant to provide a plausible context.

The official purpose of the simulation was to coordinate hospital services in the management of patients with influenza-like illness. Eighty actors playing patients came in through the front door of the hospital and were sent to different departments depending on their symptoms (pulmonary conditions, tuberculosis, etc.). Twenty 'players' treated them in the services, and two 'simulators' communicated with other hospitals on a hotline. Those diagnosed with H5N1 were evacuated by ambulance through the back door of the hospital, where the media took pictures. The head of the Department of Health gave a press conference after visiting the hospital but the journalists asked him about a new bacterium found in a private jacuzzi, not about the exercise itself. The drill's success was not questioned; it was deemed successful because it had been held. The scenario was designed in such a way that no surprising event could happen: the only reality that came up was the bacteria in the jacuzzi, not the virus in bird markets. What is considered as a difficult task in times of crisis – the triage of patients with pandemic flu who must be separated to avoid contamination and will receive emergency treatment (Nguyen 2010; Redfield 2013) – was managed in the scenario as a routine operation.

The widespread generalisation of simulation exercises for epidemic preparedness has made it almost impossible to track. In the case of the African continent, which holds a special place on the global health security map as a hotspot of emergence and as a terrain of failed governance and political instability, the first wave of simulation exercises was implemented in the wake of the avian flu crisis (which hit wild birds and poultry in Nigeria and Cameroon as well as Egypt) as part of the pandemic influenza preparedness plans requested by the WHO through the 2005 revision of the International Health Regulations (IHR). These first exercises notably aimed at bringing together human and animal health services and professionals under the emerging One Health paradigm. Increasing terrorist threats in Africa also led most African states to use the technique to address this risk, making it familiar to most governments. But the use of simulation exercises became epidemic in the post-Ebola context, when a series of international initiatives such as the US-led Global Health Security Agenda energetically sought to build an infrastructure of preparedness, epidemic surveillance, and outbreak response. From Maputo to Dakar, the simulation of epidemics has become a pre-packaged, standardised, normative exercise, with measurable and reportable outputs and indicators.

The standardisation of epidemic scenarios, which is stressed by the organisers of simulations as a way to mitigate the threat of panic by producing automatised behaviours, leads us to propose a hypothesis on the emergence of these epidemic scenarios. It is striking that simulation has also developed during the twentieth century in surgery as a technique to intervene in patients' bodies with standardised gestures to control human emotions in the confrontation with disease. Epidemiology and surgery were fostered by the experience of the First World War, but it is only at the end of the century with the possibilities opened by digitalization to follow a disease in the globe or in the body on a screen that simulate invaded hospitals as a technique of disease management. Sham surgery has developed as a fake medical intervention that mimics the therapeutic effects and could be considered as an equivalent of placebo in clinical trials. Since surgeons and hospital managers have to take difficult decisions faced with unpredictable diseases, the aim of simulations is to reduce the uncertainty by producing in the individual body and in the collective team standardised habits. The military origins of this idea are obvious, although we have little documentation so far on the transfer of simulation techniques from the army to public health.

Realism and its critiques

Another common trait between simulations of epidemics and the use of simulation in surgery is the introduction of mannequins who play the role of fake patients to trigger adapted behaviours. Historian Tracy Davis has showed that techniques invented by the world of Civil Defence in the United States and the United Kingdom after 1945 came directly from the world of theatre. 'Theater (and not merely spectacle)', she argues, 'had a utility in twentieth-century governance, education and social life, central not only to how anxiety was expressed, but more importantly to how people envisioned ways to identify and resolve anxious problems' (Davis 2007: 4). Exercises were also organised to simulate a nuclear explosion using animals as surrogates to study the outdoor impact of radiation (Masco 2006). Simulation designers in civil defence were therefore less concerned with the participation of the public than with the realism of the artefacts composing a world in which the coming catastrophe seems to be realised – what is called in the language of theatre 'accessories'.

As early as 1964, the US Army had standardised a 'Casualty Simulation Kit', also known as Device 11E10, to help produce 'realistic wounds' for disaster-response simulation exercises. An early instance of the military-humanitarian kit (Redfield 2013), the case contained ready-to-use make-up, bandages, and tags. 'Realism, the user's manual stated, is essential' (Armed Forces Institute of Pathology 1964). In the same vein, Sandrine Revet (2013) has studied how simulations of earthquakes in Lima, Peru play on the use of make-up to produce an effect of real wounds so as to engage the actors in the simulation. Similarly, organisers of epidemic simulations are very concerned with the objects which instantiate the reality of the epidemic and circulate between the different stages of simulations.

During Exercise Redwood in Hong Kong, actors who played patients wore tags around their necks indicating their symptoms as well as their name, address, nationality, sex, and age. These cards were red or green to indicate whether they had the flu or only influenza-like illness. They did not have to fake being sick; their only role was to move to the designated departments. In another exercise organised by the Centre for Health Protection, a plane was evacuated because a patient had been found with influenza-like illness; those who sat next to the patient received a red tag, and those who sat at a good distance received a yellow tag. Interestingly, the actors playing patients with influenza-like illness came from a humanitarian association, the Auxiliary Medical Service (AMS). During their own exercises, performed every month, they train how to rescue victims of car accidents or fires, simulating heartbeats on dummies with fake hearts. Tags have an indirect effect of reality as bearers of signs, while dummies can actually simulate the heartbeat of an injured victim. It can be said, consequently, that when they simulate patients wearing tags and caps in an epidemic exercise, members of the AMS literally act as if they were dummies. There is a fundamental distinction in real ground exercises between actors and players. While actors are passive, reduced to the artefacts that 'act' or 'speak for them', simulators are active, since they can introduce uncertainty by the way they combine these artefacts in the scenario. If actors have to appear 'real' to produce good images in the media, simulators introduce variations at the virtual level in the situations proposed by the scenario. The 'reluctant patient' is thus a variation within the scenario to surprise other actors and force them to act as if the scene was real: in order to avoid routine and standardisation, simulators introduce 'the reluctant patient' as a standardised tool of de-standardisation – or as an active actor to shake the habits of passive actors.

It is interesting to notice that chickens slaughtered in the scenario were not conceived as 'reluctant patients' but only as figurants in the script or as plants in the decorum. Because chickens are regularly culled in the Central Market of Hong Kong when they are suspected to carry influenza viruses, employees of the Agriculture Department don't have to simulate a slaughter to know how to manipulate carcasses. By contrast, in Singapore, where bird flu has never been found, employees of slaughterhouses regularly practice simulations of outbreaks on chickens imported alive from Malaysia. In Taiwan, endangered wild birds are the actors of exercises of vaccination under the guise of mannequins or decoys (Keck 2018). It can be argued, therefore, that chickens remain at the margins of the simulation while the reluctant patient is put at the centre of the stage – with regular actors populating the stage and simulators remaining off-stage.

The anthropology of ritual has recently argued that standardised repetition of action with a strong emotional investment should not be analysed as forms of dissimulation (of a truth that should be revealed by the ethnographer) but as forms of simulation (of an uncertainty on the future that is shared by the ethnographer) (Houseman 2002; Hamayon 2015) which brings ritual closer to a public play with social identities rather than to the religious disclosure of a secret perceived as sacred (Gusterson 1996). This idea is useful to analyse the shift of identifications on the stage of simulation as different ways to relate to future pandemics. If the reality of the epidemic is contested by critical actors it is because there are different ways to engage in social activities and justify one's behaviour in collective frameworks (Boltanski 2011).

The question of realism and reality during simulation exercises raises another set of issues. Simulations can never fully assume that the real is kept at a controlled distance (through the techniques of realism): the real may return during the simulation, at any moment and under surprising forms. Echoing Jean Baudrillard's (1994) thought experiment about a fake hold-up organised with fake weapons, where the fake gangsters could be exposed to very real consequences, obtaining real money or being shot at with real bullets, such returns or leaks of the real are classic features of simulation exercises. In her work on the simulation of aggressions during self-defence classes for women in Egypt, Perrine Lachenal (2014) has shown how the (male) instructor could inflict real pain, real wounds, and real humiliation to (female) participants, so as to train them to the realistic conditions of a potential street incident. This led to situations of unease and conflicts during simulations, showing precisely that the distinction between a simulated and a real aggression may be less obvious that the device of the simulation exercise assumed.

Another example can be drawn from a large-scale simulation of a flood in the rural town of Boromo in Burkina Faso, organised in April 2009 by the governmental committee for emergency relief (CONASUR). A fake refugee camp for the victims was organised and according to the scenario, 500 actors were sheltered there with access to food, water, and basic services. The journalist who covered the exercise noted that at the health centre of the camp the medical teams were quickly overwhelmed: they 'saw the simulated medical consultations transform very rapidly into real consultations' as the actors took advantage of the situation to talk with a real doctor. 'We recorded 139 patients', explained Dr Seydou Ouattara, 'it went beyond the exercise. Among these patients, some were injured on the site of the exercises, others had headaches; most were chronic diseases' (Anonymous 1). In addition, the 518 actors, representing 101 households according the scenario, received real 30 kg rice bags. Not only the simulation got caught 'unwittingly' into the real, but it also offered journalists and audiences a glimpse of the state of need of the local populations – it was a device of revelation that challenged paradoxically, as real patients queued at fake medical posts, the prioritisation of disaster preparedness over more classic public health or development interventions. And when real flooding occurred in the region in September the same year and demonstrated not only the government's unpreparedness but its sheer absence (President Compaoré was in Libya celebrating Gaddafi's birthday), the newspaper Bendré noted that the money (200 million CFA Francs; 300,000 Euros) spent by the CONASUR on simulating them five months earlier could have been better spent: 'one does not throw so much money for not existing' (Anonymous 2).

Another example from Cameroon: on September 13, 2017 a press release from the Ministry of Health began to circulate on social networks, announcing nine cases of cholera in the city of Douala. As often in Cameroon, 'radio-trottoir' followed, spreading the rumour across the city, and 'panic' set in, according to the local journalists (Anonymous 3). Health workers had not seen single case, though: the press release had actually leaked from a simulation exercise organised the same week with an official closure ceremony organised in a prestigious hotel of Yaoundé. The simulation, this time, had leaked onto the real. In a strange looping effect, the false alert was produced by the very preparedness apparatus that was supposed to deal with it.

Such events are reminders that what constitutes reality is never a given, or at least that some situations are undecidably ambiguous, especially in contexts where simulation (in the sense of deception, parody, and falsification) has a long history as a political technique. In Cameroon where post-colonial governmentality resembles more an 'unusual and grotesque art of representation' (Mbembe 2001: 114) than calculated biopolitics, the remark must be taken seriously. For example, the popular conclusion about two famous episodes of nationwide rumours about the president Paul Biya's death in a Swiss hospital was that the President had actually started the rumour himself by simulating its own death to test experimentally the loyalty of its supporters and inner circles – the simulation again as a way to reveal the true reality.

Conclusion: simulation as a technique of non-government

Global health has been analysed by some observers as marking the end of sovereign states replaced by NGOs, international organisations (WHO, OIE, FAO), and private foundations (such as the Gates Foundation) in the funding of public health interventions. However, simulations of epidemics have been appropriated by national states to display their sovereignty on a territory threatened by a pathogen coming from abroad. It can be argued, therefore, that simulation is not the end of the sovereign State but a cosmetic transformation to make it more acceptable following global standards. As they offer a playing ground where the compliance to international norms can be assessed, simulation exercises can also be seen from the perspective of a continent known for its bewildering capacity to adopt, appropriate, and eventually empty out global norms (Mbembe 2001; Ferguson 2006) as possible objects of mimicry. The lack of engagement of actors was suggested for example by the ironic remarks of one participant in an avian flu simulation exercise conducted in 2008 in a luxury hotel of Douala, Cameroon (Lachenal 2015): 'We gathered, we took the pictures, we sent them to the WHO, and that's it!'. Just as any other ritual of global governance, simulation exercises may be staged (and nothing more than staged) thus opening the possibility of *a simulation of the simulation.*

Simulation allows public health actors to perform the State even though they know that it can be criticised for its lack of action. In situations of limited resources the state requires individuals to perform situations it doesn't have the capacity to cope with. Simulation of the capacity to govern may thus be the mode of existence of the neo-liberal state, which is also characterised more generally by the importance of public performances, simulations, and spectacle. Jean and John Comaroff, in their study of the simulations of accidents by the South African police, stated that exercises of simulation take a positive function in the postcolony: that of a 'simulacrum of governance, a rite staged to make actual and authoritative, at least in the eyes of an executive bureaucracy, the activity of those responsible for law and order, and by extension, to enact the very possibility of governement' (Comaroff 2006: 289). Seen in this light, such simulations of epidemics could appear as rituals staged to regenerate the very idea of national public health when few would believe in the capacity of the state to implement any public health policy.

By contrast with African neo-liberal states, Hong Kong reveals another transition from colonial to neo-liberal governance. In the 1960s, the British government reinforced its public health policy in hospitals and markets as a way to respond to the threat of strikes coming from Communist China; for a short period a welfare state was developed in the colony to avoid its collapse into the socialist block (Caroll 2007). However, since the 1997 handover to China, the Hong Kong government has followed the liberal traditions of the British colony and intervenes the least possible in the flows of commodities, persons, and finance that circulate on its territory in order to maintain its position as a hub between China and the rest of the world. But the security of its population – Hong Kong citizens, Chinese wealthy immigrants, Western expatriates – is a great concern under threats of influenza coming from Chinese birds along with other environmental damages of the Chinese industrial growth. Simulations of avian influenza are therefore key instruments for the government to show its willingness to protect its population. Hence the creation of the Centre for Health Protection as a reactive agency communicating immediately in case of an outbreak and organising simulations to anticipate future outbreaks. Due to its position as 'Asia's world city', Hong Kong has focused the main characteristics of exercises organised in the Asia-Pacific region and oriented them toward its specific situation on the border with China.

Cases of simulations of epidemics from Africa and Asia show that the proliferation of exercises based on worst-case scenarios led to a confusion between simulation and reality. It doesn't mean that reality has become virtual, as is often criticised in social descriptions of simulation, but that reality has been designed through a form of justification adequate to neo-liberal societies. When simulations are made 'realistic', it means that reality must be conceived as a test for the capacity of the state to govern its population. When the state renounces investing in the public health infrastructures that guarantee the stability of the social world (for instance, which pathogens are considered dangerous, and how to treat them), it can only multiply exercises for pathogens that will emerge anytime from anywhere. Every public health crisis is thus a test for the capacity of governments to react and for its agents to save lives, almost on the same level as tests passed by ordinary citizens to show their capacity to govern themselves. In a public health system where crisis is the permanent condition and emergency the dominant affect, simulation is a way to test its actors for the competences they have developed in coping with emerging infectious diseases and other threats of social life.

Acknowledgements

Frédéric Keck and Guillaume Lachenal acknowledge the project Simulations supervised by Sandrine Revet at Sciences-Po Paris.

References

Abraham, Thomas *Twenty-First Century Plague: The Story of SARS, with a New Preface on Avian Flu* (Hong Kong: Hong Kong University Press, 2007).

Adams, Vincanne, Maureen Murphy, and Adele Clarke 'Anticipation: Technoscience, life, affect, temporality', *Subjectivity* 28 (1) (2009), 248–265.

Anonymous 1 'Plan de contingences multirisques et de réponses aux catastrophes. Le Burkina teste ses capacités à travers une simulation à Boromo', *L'opinion* (April 2009). www.zedcom.bf/quoti/act128.php

Anonymous 2 'Confidentiel 561', *Bendré* (September 14, 2009). www.journalbendre.net/spip.php?article2963

Anonymous 3 'Cameroun – Santé: Un exercice de routine créé une fausse alerte à l'épidémie de choléra à Douala', *Actus du Cameroun* (September 15, 2017). https://actucameroun.com/2017/09/15/cameroun-sante-exercice-de-routine-cree-fausse-alerte-a-lepidemie-de-cholera-a-douala/

Armed Forces Institute of Pathology, U.S.A. *Instructor's Guide for Casualty Simulation Kit Device 11E10* (Washington D.C., 1964).

Armstrong, Melanie 'Rehearsing for the plague: Citizens, security, and simulation', *Canadian Review of American Studies* 42 (1) (2012), 105–120.

Baudrillard, Jean *Simulacra and Simulation* (Ann Arbor: University of Michigan Press, 1994).

Boltanski, Luc *On Critique: A Sociology of Emancipation* (Cambridge: Polity Press, 2011).

Brown, David 'How computer modelers took on the Ebola outbreak' (2015). https://spec trum.ieee.org/computing/software/how-computer-modelers-took-on-the-ebola-outbreak

Caduff, Carlo *The Pandemic Perhaps: Dramatic Events in a Public Culture of Danger* (Oakland: University of California Press, 2015).

Caroll, John M *A Concise History of Hong Kong* (Hong Kong: Hong Kong University Press, 2007).

Chakrabarty, Dipesh *Provincializing Europe: Postcolonial Thought and Historical Difference* (Princeton, NJ: Princeton University Press, 2000).

Collier, Stephen, and Andrew Lakoff 'Vital systems security: Reflexive biopolitics and the government of emergency', *Theory Culture and Society* 32 (2) (2015), 19–51.

Comaroff, Jean, and John L. Comaroff 'Criminal obsessions, after Foucault: Postcoloniality, policing and the metaphysics of disorder', In Jean Comaroff, and John L. Comaroff (eds.), *Law and Disorder in the Postcolony*, pp. 273–298 (Chicago, IL: The University of Chicago Press, 2006).

Davis, Tracy *Stages of Emergency: Cold War Nuclear Civil Defense* (Durham, NC: Duke University Press, 2007).

Diamond, Jared *Guns, Germs and Steel: The Fates of Human Societies* (New York: W. W. Norton & Company, 1997).

Faria N.R., J. Quick, I.M. Claro, J. Thézé, J. G. de Jesus, M. Giovanetti, M.U.G. Kraemer 'Establishment and cryptic transmission of Zika virus in Brazil and the Americas', *Nature* 546 (7658) (2017), 406–410.

Ferguson, James *Global Shadows: Africa in the Neoliberal World Order* (Durham, DC: Duke University Press, 2006).

Galison Peter 'The future of scenarios: State science fiction', In Bolette Blaagaard, and Iris van der Tuin (eds.), *The Subject of Rosi Braidotti: Politics and Concepts*, pp. 38–46 (London and New York: Bloomsbury Academic, 2014).

Ghamari-Tabrizi, Sharon *The Worlds of Herman Kahn: The Intuitive Science of Thermonuclear War* (Cambridge, MA: Harvard University Press, 2005).

Giles-Vernick, Tamara, and Susan Craddock, eds. *Influenza and Public Health: Learning from Past Pandemics* (London: Routledge and Earthscan, 2010).

Giles-Vernick, Tamara, Ch Didier Gondola, Guillaume Lachenal, and William H. Schneider 'Social history, biology and the emergence of HIV in colonial Africa', *Journal of African History* 54 (1) (2013), 11–30.

Gusterson, Hugh *Nuclear Rites: A Weapons Laboratory at the End of the Cold War* (Stanford, CA: Stanford University Press, 1996).

Hamayon, Roberte *Why We Play: An Anthropological Study* (Chicago, IL: The University of Chicago Press, 2015).

Hamblin, Jacob D. *Arming Mother Nature: The Birth of Environmental Catastrophism* (Oxford: Oxford University Press, 2013).

Hanoun, Claude 'La grippe', In *Encyclopédie Médico-Chirurgicale*, Vol. 8 (Paris: Elsevier-Masson, 1993).

Houseman, Michael 'Dissimulation and simulation as modes of religious reflexivity', *Social Anthropology* 10 (1) (2002), 77–89.

Humphries, Mark Osborne 'Paths of infection: The first world war and the origins of the 1918 influenza pandemic', *War in History* 21 (1) (2014), 55–81.

Kahn, Hermann *Thinking About the Unthinkable* (Princeton, NJ: Princeton University Press, 1962).

Keck, Frédéric 'Avian preparedness. Simulations of bird diseases in reverse scenarios of extinction in Hong Kong, Taiwan and Singapore', *The Journal of the Royal Anthropological Institute* N.S 24 (2) (2018), 330–347.

King, Nicholas 'Security, disease, commerce: Ideologies of postcolonial global health', *Social Studies of Science* 32 (5–6) (2002), 763–789.

King, Nicholas 'The scale politics of emerging diseases', *Osiris* 19 (2004), 62–70.

Kupperman, Richard H. 'Vulnerable America', In R. James Woolsey (ed.), *Nuclear Arms: Ethics, Strategy, Politics*, pp. 570–580 (San Francisco: Institute for Contemporary Studies Press, 1983).

Lachenal, Guillaume 'Outbreak of unknown origin in the Tripoint Zone', *Limn* (5) (2014), epub. http://limn.it/outbreak-of-unknown-origin-in-the-tripoint-zone/

Lachenal, Guillaume 'Lessons in medical nihilism. Virus hunters, neoliberalism and the AIDS crisis in Cameroon', In Wenzel Geissler (ed.), *Science and the Parastate in Africa*, pp. 103–141 (Durham, NC: Duke University Press, 2015).

Lachenal, Perrine *Self-défense féminine dans le Caire en révolution: Techniques du genre et jeux de violence*. Thèse de doctorat en Anthropologie, Université d'Aix-Marseille, 2014.

Lakoff, Andrew *Unprepared: Global Health in a Time of Emergency* (Oakland: University of California Press, 2017).

Mackenzie, Adrian 'Bringing sequences to life. How Bioinformatics corporealizes sequence data', *New Genetics and Society* 22 (3) (2003), 315–332.

MacPhail, Teresa *Viral Network. A Pathography of the H1N1 Influenza Pandemic* (Ithaca: Cornell University Press, 2014).

Masco, Joseph *The Nuclear Borderlands: The Manhattan Project in Post-Cold War New Mexico* (Princeton, NJ: Princeton University Press, 2006).

Manson, Elisabeth. *Infectious Change: Reinventing Chinese Public Health After and Epidemic* (Stanford, CA: Stanford University Press, 2016).

Mbembe, J. Achille *On the Postcolony* (Berkeley, CA and London: The University of California Press, 2001).

MSF *Ebola: Pushed to the Limit and Beyond* (2015). www.msf.org/ebola-pushed-limit-and-beyond

Nguyen, Vinh-Kim *The Republic of Therapy: Triage and Sovereignty in West Africa's Time of AIDS* (Durham, NC: Duke University Press, 2010).

Pepin, Jacques *The Origins of AIDS* (Cambridge: Cambridge University Press, 2011).

Preston, Richard *The Hot Zone* (New York: Random House, 1994).

Preston, Richard *The Cobra Event* (New York: Random House, 1998).

Redfield, Peter *Life in Crisis: The Ethical Journey of Doctors Without Borders* (Berkeley, CA: The University of California Press, 2013).

Revet, Sandrine ' "A small world": Ethnography of a natural disaster simulation in Lima, Peru', *Social Anthropology/Anthropologie Sociale* 21 (1) (2013), 38–53.

Samimian-Darash, Limor 'Practicing uncertainty: Scenario-based preparedness exercises in Israel', *Cultural Anthropology* 31 (3) (2016), 359–386.

Schull, Natasha 'The Gaming of chance: Online poker software and the potentialization of uncertainty', In Samimian-Darash Limor, and Rabinow Paul (eds.), *Modes of Uncertainty: Anthropological Cases*, pp. 46–66 (Chicago, IL: The University of Chicago Press, 2015).

Shortridge, Kennedy F., and Charles H. Stuart-Harris 'An influenza epicentre?' *Lancet* ii (1982), 812–813.

Sismondo, Sergio 'Models, simulations and their objects', *Science in Context* 12 (2) (1999), 247–60.

Smith, G., X. H. Fan, J. Wang, K. S. Li, K. Qin, J. X. Zhang, D. Vijaykrishna, C. L. Cheung, K. Huang, J. M. Rayner, J. S. M. Peiris, H. Chen, R. G. Webster, and Y. Guan 'Emergence and predominance of an H5N1 influenza variant in China', *PNAS* 103 (45) (2006), 16936–16941.

Smith, Gavin J.D., Dhanasekaran Vijaykrishna, Justin Bahl, Samantha J. Lycett, Michael Worobey, Oliver G. Pybus, Siu Kit Ma, et al. 'Origins and evolutionary genomics of the 2009 swine-origin H1N1 Influenza A epidemic', *Nature* 459 (2009), 1122–1125.

Sunstein, Carl R. *Worst-Case Scenarios* (Cambridge, MA: Harvard University Press, 2007).

Taubenberger, Jeffery K., and D. M. Morens '1918 influenza: The mother of all pandemics', *Emerging Infectious Diseases* 12 (1) (2006), 15–22.

United Nations System Influenza Coordination *Simulation Exercises on Influenza Pandemic Responses in the Asia-Pacific Region* (Geneva, 2008).

Wolfe, Nathan, Claire Dunavan, and Jared Diamond 'Origins of major human infectious diseases', *Nature* 447 (2007), 279–283.

Yong, Ed. 'What Bill Gates fears most', *The Atlantic* (April 27, 2018). www.theatlantic.com/science/archive/2018/04/what-bill-gates-fears-most/559007/

Zylberman, Patrick *Tempêtes microbiennes: Essai sur la politique de sécurité sanitaire dans le monde transatlantique* (Paris: Gallimard, 2013).

2   Great anticipations*

Carlo Caduff

[E]ach catastrophe is somehow new despite its repetitiveness.

Mary Ann Doane

1

Let me start this piece with a series of headlines:

Is bird flu the next pandemic?
(*National Geographic*, December 2004)

What will the next influenza pandemic look like?
(*Scientific American*, September 2011)

How one scientist is preventing the next pandemic
(*Time*, October 2011)

Where will the next pandemic come from?
(*Wall Street Journal*, October 2011)

Anticipating the next pandemic
(*New York Times*, September 2012)

Is this the next pandemic?
(*The Guardian*, March 2013)

Stopping the next pandemic today
(*Washington Post*, June 2015)

The next pandemic could be dripping on your head
(*National Public Radio*, February 2017)

How to prepare for the next pandemic
(*New Scientist*, February 2017)

DOI: 10.4324/9780429461897-3

The world is not ready for the next pandemic
(*Time*, May 2017)

Where will the next pandemic come from?
(*Wall Street Journal*, June 2017)

The next pandemic may come from bats
(*Salon*, June 2017)

Is it possible to predict the next pandemic?
(*The Atlantic*, October 2017)

With Mary Anne Doane, we might say that each headline is 'somehow new despite its repetitiveness' (Doane 2006) (p. 264). But what exactly makes a head-line somehow new?

2

The mass media fascination with mass death and mass disease has a long history, to be sure, but there is something more specific that needs to be said about the way in which viruses are going viral today (Warner 2002). What makes a disease communicable in our culture of media? To address this question, we need to take into account what Doane has said about mass media more generally: such media incessantly take 'as [their] own subject matter the documentation and revalida-tion of [their] own discursive problematic' (Doane 2006) (p. 253). In this chapter, I argue that the mass media has found in the idea of the next pandemic an ideal opportunity to corroborate its own discursive problematic.

What is the mass media's discursive problematic? Focusing on the nineteenth-century detective novel, Franco Moretti identified a norm, which is at the heart of mass media communication more generally: 'It must tell ever-new stories because it moves within the culture of the novel, which always demands new content; and at the same time it must reproduce a scheme which is always the same' (Moretti 1983) (p. 141). The permanent production of novelty is at the heart of mass media communication. In the global health concern with emerging infectious diseases the mass media has found a powerful resource for such novelty. Indeed, the trope of the next pandemic has become an important location for the production of con-tent that is 'new despite its repetitiveness' (Doane 2006) (p. 264).

Today's mass media fascination with the next pandemic is partly due to the fact that it operates as corroboration of the mass media's own discursive problematic: the necessity of creating and maintaining a constant sense of newness. The func-tion of mass media communication, according to Niklas Luhmann, is to simulta-neously 'generate and process irritation' (Luhmann 2000) (p. 22).[1] Invested in the production, circulation, and consumption of irritation, mass media communica-tion stimulates 'the constantly renewed willingness to be prepared for surprises'.

The trope of the next pandemic, in this sense, is a fertile ground for the mass media and its discursive problematic.

This piece examines the permanent production of novelty and the continuous communication of discontinuity as a paradoxical feature of mass media communication. The observation that mass media communication is fuelling fears about a coming global health catastrophe raises a number of questions: What happens with pandemic influenza once it becomes an occasion for mass media to document and revalidate their own discursive problematic? What are the consequences for other infectious diseases such as Ebola and Zika? Doane has shown why and how mass media are compelled by the catastrophic in general, but in this chapter, I examine one articulation of the catastrophic, tracing the shape pandemic influenza takes in our culture of media.

Empirically the chapter follows a series of articles published in prominent newspapers and magazines. Of anthropological interest is not the content, which has a purely quantitative function (it literally 'fills' the page), but the form of the discourse.[2] The perspective presented in this chapter reveals four formal characteristics. Today's mass media discourse about the next pandemic uses objective proclamations; it promotes its own consumption; it prevents the formation of a historical consciousness; it is incapable of closure.

3

In July 2005, Michael Osterholm, Director of the Center for Infectious Disease Research and Policy at the University of Minnesota, published an article in *Foreign Affairs*, an influential US magazine. The piece came with the following title: 'Preparing for the next pandemic' (Osterholm 2005). It stated: 'Influenza pandemics have posed the greatest threat of a worldwide calamity caused by infectious disease'. Drawing attention to the spread of avian flu in Asia, Osterholm suggested that a pandemic was imminent. 'The reality of a coming pandemic . . . cannot be avoided', he wrote. 'Only its impact can be lessened'. A global pandemic 'would trigger a reaction that would change the world overnight', warned Osterholm. The consequences would be catastrophic.

> Foreign trade and travel would be reduced or even ended in an attempt to stop the virus from entering new countries – even though such efforts would probably fail given the infectiousness of influenza and the volume of illegal crossings that occur at most borders. It is likely that transportation would also be significantly curtailed domestically, as smaller communities sought to keep the disease contained.

Fear, panic, and chaos would be the inevitable result. 'Military leaders would have to develop strategies to defend the country and also protect against domestic insurgency with armed forces that would likely be compromised by the disease'. Meanwhile, the global economy 'would shut down'. It was time to take the threat seriously and launch a public health campaign to prevent the worst.

'Even if an H5N1 pandemic is a year away, the world must plan for the same problems with the same fervor', wrote Osterholm in his article.

> Major campaigns must be initiated to prepare the nonmedical and medical sectors. Pandemic planning must be on the agenda of every school board, manufacturing plant, investment firm, mortuary, state legislature, and food distributor in the United States and beyond. There is an urgent need to reassess the vulnerability of the global economy to ensure that surges in demand can be met. Critical heath-care and consumer products and commodities must be stockpiled. Health professionals must learn how to better communicate risk and must be able to both provide the facts and acknowledge the unknowns to a frightened or panicked population.

For Osterholm living in the present meant living in anticipation of the catastrophic event. His aim was to convince public health professionals to perceive the present as a momentary suspension before the next pandemic struck. How much time before it occurred? How much time was left to prepare? Attuned to the temporal imperatives of pandemic preparedness, Osterhom warned: 'A pandemic is coming. . . . It could happen tonight, next year, or even ten years from now. . . . Time is running out to prepare for the next pandemic'.

As a professor at the University of Minnesota, a member of the prestigious Institute of Medicine of the National Academy of Science and a bestselling author, Osterholm is a prominent figure with access to the media. Over the past decade he has become one of the nation's most outspoken public health professionals advocating substantial investments in preparedness – a concern representative of a broader global health apparatus (Caduff 2015; Lakoff 2017). To address the catastrophic event that was looming on the horizon, Osterholm founded his own research and policy agency, CIDRAP, the Center for Infectious Disease Research and Policy. CIDRAP features an online news division tasked with the publication of daily news updates on the latest disease event. Similar to the immune system, the job of the news division is to operate as a search engine.[3] It monitors global media sources on a daily basis, searching websites, news wires, and online discussion forums for important information.[4] Each 'news scan' offers a daily epidemic intelligence update on the infectious disease front. At the heart of these updates are often speculations about the future.

4

'We live in times', writes Brian Massumi, 'when what is yet to occur not only climbs to the top of the news but periodically takes blaring precedence over what has actually happened' (Massumi 2010) (see as well Massumi 2015). This focus on the future has taken a particular shape in the historical present: to prepare for what's to come is to prepare for what's next. Massumi's observation points to the emergence of a persistent demand characteristic of a modern sense of time: the demand to consider what's next. The promise, which ostensibly makes this demand optimistic, is that a consideration of the next will permit people to prepare for the future. Those who took the necessary time to make the necessary preparations are presumably more likely to survive the shock of surprise. This compulsion can take the form of optimisation: 'the moral responsibility of citizens to secure their "best possible futures"' (Adams et al. 2009).

Many scholars have examined regimes of anticipation over the past decade, but here I am concerned with the role of repetition in attempts to anticipate future events. To understand the logic of anticipation, we need to investigate the idea of the next as that which both disavows and thus makes possible repetition.[5] Instead of focusing on content (what is next?), this chapter draws attention to form; it highlights a structure (the structure of the next) and illuminates a pattern (the serial nature of the next). This shift of focus from content to form moves the scholarly discussion beyond an epistemological concern with the production of knowledge that tends to dominate in the literature (Anderson 2010; Aradau and van Munster 2011; Barker 2012; Briggs 2011; Briggs and Hallin 2016; Lakoff 2007; Lakoff 2008; Samimian-Darash 2009; Samimian-Darash 2013). Using a series of numbers to present a series of insights, this chapter imitates the form that is under examination.

What, then, is the next? The next figures in the now not simply as an index of the future. The next is imagined in a particular way: it's what's immediately following or succeeding; it's what's coming after in a series or sequence of potentially surprising events. But the next has not only a temporal meaning. What's next is near in place and close at hand. Thus, the next has a distinct spatial and temporal meaning, which makes it different from the more general idea of the future (which may be far away). The next, by contrast, is next. It's near, it's close, it's next.

Let's move on to the next then.

5

What will you do when the next strikes? You need to already know how to respond when it happens. In the United States, government officials suggested that simulations, exercises, and drills represented essential techniques enabling the now to prepare for the next. Continuing participation in preparedness activities allowed individuals, communities, and companies to be near to what's near and close to what's close. Borrowed from the military, officials promoted these activities as contribution to the development of embodied dispositions, making the response to the next a matter not of contemplation and reflection, but of instinct and habit (Caduff 2015; Lakoff 2008; Masco 2014). From the perspective of preparedness, the next was preparable but not preventable. According to experts, the catastrophic event was unavoidable; the question was not whether it would happen, but how to respond to it when it happens.

At the core of an expanding series of simulations, exercises, and drills for imagined events was the cybernetic vision of a nation ready for the next, a nation permanently preparing for discontinuity – that is, living in preparedness. What Luhmann identified as essential function of mass media – to constantly renew the willingness to be prepared for surprises – is also at the heart of preparedness and its key message: expect the unexpected. Preparedness for catastrophic events is not just a response to the experience of catastrophic events; it is also a response to the experience of the world as endless series of news, an experience that the mass media created.

6

Are you prepared for what's next?

7

Off to the next.

8

In March 2007, Osterholm, the public health professional who claims to be near to what's near and close to what's close, published an update in *Foreign Affairs*. 'The facts remain incontrovertible', he declared in his piece 'Unprepared for a pandemic' (Osterholm 2007). 'Like earthquakes, hurricanes, and tsunamis, influenza pandemics are recurring natural disasters'. And so there was no doubt that a pandemic would happen. 'No one can predict when the next pandemic will occur or how severe it will be', he said. 'But it will occur for sure, and because of the interdependence of the global economy today, its implications will reach far beyond its toll on human health'. To concretise the certainty of impending calamity, he offered evidence that could not be ignored: scientists were discovering more and more genetic changes in the avian influenza virus. The microbe was mutating, infecting more and more animals and more and more humans, making it, in the expert's view, the 'likely strain of the next pandemic'.[6]

Yet preparedness for the next pandemic had not made sufficient progress in the United States. 'The issue has generated only limited attention in both the public and the private sectors . . . because preparing for a pandemic is a daunting challenge to begin with and because disaster has not yet struck'. But the fact that the inevitable had yet to occur was no excuse for the lack of immediate action. 'The opportunity to save millions of lives cannot be passed up. Even if such efforts come too late to stave off the next pandemic, at least they would help in the one after that', wrote Osterholm.

9

The next can strike anywhere, at any time.

10

The next: closer than you think.

11

In May 2013, Osterholm was back in the news with an update on the next. 'The next contagion: Closer than you think', was the title of Osterholm's editorial in the opinion pages of the *New York Times*. Invoking an ongoing outbreak of avian influenza in China, the public health expert identified a new, 'and far more widespread, ailment that has gotten little attention: *contagion exhaustion*'. The constant stream of updates had led people to ignore recent developments and dismiss warnings about an impending calamity. In his piece, Osterholm addressed a key problem of mass media communication: how to make sure that the continuity of the communication is not undermining the discontinuity of the content. Had the permanent reproduction of newness exhausted the novelty of the new? What happens when repetition of the message increasingly threatens the possibility of surprise? Had the constant focus on the next lost its mobilising power?

Officials at the Centers for Disease Control and Prevention (CDC) were also worried about the fading interest in preparedness for the next pandemic. 'If the pandemic doesn't hit soon', an official told me, 'public interest is going to wane, congressional interest is going to wane, and we will lose the momentum because we will probably end up losing a lot of the funding, and we will lose the visibility, and we will lose the priority and status that we have'. The official went on, 'We tend to be complacent, we go back, we put our guards down. Unfortunately, I think this country has to go through a series of events in order to be at the level that it should be in order to respond and effectively recover'.

Struggling against the loss of interest in the next pandemic, Osterholm emphasised the stakes. He argued that the toll would be economic and not just human:

> Studies have shown that a severe global pandemic, caused by viruses like influenza . . ., could bring the global economy . . . to its knees. When people are too sick or too afraid to work, borders are closed and global supply chains break, and trade falls. Over months, the economic costs could send the world into recession.

In today's world, a pandemic would bring the global economy to a halt. Avian influenza may seem far away in China, but tomorrow it 'could be at America's doorstep'. What was happening now in China could be next in America.

12

The next: Not a question of if, but when.

13

I waited for the next attack, and the next after that.[7]

14

In the world of preparedness, each event appears as an episode, a variation of something that has already happened in the past and that will happen again in the future. However, with the exception of preparedness as constantly renewed willingness to prepare for the next (and the next after that), there is no overarching framework that would connect the series of events over time. The lack of a larger framework has profound consequences. Conventional narrative seriality defers the moment of closure. But this deferral of closure is precisely what enables people to expect an end. The lack of an overarching story that would connect the series of events is essential because it destroys the very possibility of entertaining the sense of an ending.[8] In the world of preparedness, it has become impossible to even conceive of the possibility of an end. The next can always extend itself, and move on to the next next.

15

After the next, there is always the next after that.

16

An orientation, which looks out toward the next, will always look out toward the next next (and the next after that). This potentially endless extension of the next remits it to the strange space/time of the after: the next comes after itself, both in relation to a past next and in relation to a future next. The next chases itself; it is after itself.[9]

17

The next is next, no matter what.

18

The next contains within itself a constant return to and renewal of itself.

19

The constant release of updates makes people constantly and continuously expect a sequel. These sequels seem to follow one another in a series. What the idea of the next introduces into the political imaginary of our time is a sense of seriality.

20

Serialisation is a fundamental feature of modern mass production. When the mass media appropriated serialisation in the nineteenth century, people learned to expect a sequel. Dickens's *Great Expectations* was a striking success, not least because the author managed to publish the novel in weekly instalments. At the time of the first edition, the publication of the novel progressed in parallel to the development of the story. The suspension of the novel's publication was simultaneously a suspension of the narrative. While the suspension of the publication created expectations of continuity, the suspension of the narrative created expectations of closure. For the reader, the promise of continuity came with the promise of conclusion – of learning how the story ends.[10] Yet the end of the story was also potentially a frustration for the reader's desire, a desire stimulated by constant delays and deferrals. What the mass culture of modern capitalism detected in techniques of strategic interruption – ideally at moments of great narrative tension – was the possibility of drawing readers into the temporal unfolding of the narrative itself (Wu 2016). Delays and deferrals contributed to the expansion of the market for novels by virtue of incomplete narratives, discontinued stories that called for continuation. Such stories attached readers to the next.

The fragmented nature of a publication released in regular instalments reveals its material existence as a commodity, a commodity promoting its own consumption. The material fragmentation of the commodity extended the time of its consumption, and thus its commercial value (Hagedorn 1995). Moreover, each instalment was also a new beginning. 'We shall keep perpetually going on beginning again, regularly', declared Dickens at the end of an instalment of the *Pickwick Papers* (Hayward). Each episode offered the opportunity of continuing *and* starting again.

As a form of suspension, serialisation is a manipulation of time. It is a mediation of experience, a transformation of human sense perception, which has profound implications for subjects of desire in economies of mass production. In such economies, desire takes the form of an expectation. The purpose of an episode is to 'promote continued consumption of later episodes of the same serial'. Serials are self-promoting; they create the conditions for their own consumption.

21

In September 2014, Osterholm returned with a sequel. This time it was an epidemic of Ebola in West Africa. The disease offered an opportunity to continue and start again, with something that was new despite its repetitiveness: the next pandemic. In a *New York Times* article, Osterholm promised to reveal a dark secret: what public health professionals were afraid to say about Ebola (Osterholm 2014). 'What is not getting said publicly, despite briefings and discussions in the inner circles of the world's public health agencies', announced Osterholm, 'is that we are in totally uncharted waters and that Mother Nature is the only force in charge of the crisis at this time'. According to the public health expert, there was the possibility of a sequel to the Ebola story 'that should keep us up at night': the virus could change and become airborne. 'If certain mutations occurred, it would mean that just breathing would put one at risk of contracting Ebola'. For Osterholm, the threat of an Ebola virus transmitting rapidly through the air and not just through direct contact was real: 'until we consider it, the world will not be prepared to do what is necessary to end the epidemic'. Only the possibility of an airborne virus would force people to face the reality of the devastating epidemic and do something about it.

Experts in the United States dismissed Osterholm's speculation about an Ebola virus speeding through the air (Sifferlin 2014). 'We have observed that existing viral diseases like influenza, polio, hepatitis C and H.I.V. have not evolved to change their established route of transmission. So why does Dr Osterholm see this as a possible path for Ebola?', two microbiologists wondered. They continued: 'In our opinion, virologists are not "loath" to discuss this idea; it just seems highly improbable and, on top of that, an unproductive use of everyone's time'.

Osterholm's vision of the next was a distraction from the now. 'Raising the specter of new routes of virus transmission only distracts from the urgency of addressing what our nation and others must do to contain this Ebola outbreak'.

The CDC released an information sheet, explaining why Ebola was unlikely to become airborne. Osterholm replied that he was not concerned with what was happening now but what might happen next: 'It hasn't happened yet', he said, 'but what would happen if we had respiratory transmission?' The virus could mutate today and change into an airborne infection tomorrow. Invoking the vitality of the virus, its ability to change, Osterholm suggested that his account was inspired by the self-propelling force of the situation itself (Mayer 2013).

It was important to take the possibility seriously and 'do what we are not doing'. A massive international intervention was required. Osterholm proposed that the U.N. Security Council pass a resolution giving the United Nations 'total responsibility for controlling the outbreak, while respecting West African nations' sovereignty as much as possible'.

The Ebola virus did not mutate and become airborne. Whatever the scientific evidence for Osterholm's claims in the *New York Times*, he relied on the idea of mutation to produce another sequel and speculate one more time about the next pandemic.

22

In the world of preparedness, the present appears as a palimpsest, a page where each instance of writing amounts to an overwriting. The logic of the palimpsest refers us to a logic of spatial superimposition. The palimpsest is a layered page containing a series of subsequent episodes, where each episode is placed on top of another. All episodes are assembled on the same page, which has been overwritten and which will be overwritten, again and again, just like a newspaper website, where each day the same page will contain new content.

In the palimpsest, the now is ready to receive the next. This perception of the present as palimpsest is how the now has learned to make room for the next. Here, the subsequent is never really an extension; it is always a superimposition.

The palimpsest prevents the formation of a historical consciousness because it entails a process of systematic erasure.[11] What this erasure engenders is a fantasy, the fantasy of the blank slate. This fantasy is fundamental for any serial narration. Ruth Mayer, in her brilliant exploration of serial narration, observes how in this type of narration 'individual parts seem to follow the logic of the blank slate – every time we encounter the same cast or characters plus numerous others in the exact same basic situation that then branches out in a seemingly endless array of options'. The process of systematic erasure, which is constitutive for the palimpsest, makes it possible for individual episodes to follow a logic of return and renewal: each episode presents the same basic situation with the same basic enigma which unfolds in seemingly endless ways, before it returns to the starting point from where it will take off again. Seriality is compelling 'because it promises a perpetual renewal of the same moment', notes Mayer (2016). 'Serial figures are back again with every new installment, and they experience with great reliability the same situations and conflicts as in the first place' (Mayer 2013). The recursive process of systematic erasure, of systematic self-aggression and self-destruction, enables perpetual renewal. Episodic forms of seriality lack an overarching narrative connecting each episode. The result is not a sense of narrative progress but of 'episodic stagnation'. At the end of each episode, 'everything returns to a state of equilibrium, in which characters and setting remain unchanged' (Wu 2016). Each episode of the series contains the same scenario 'in which a conflict arises, escalates, and finally resolves itself'.

23

Season One

Season Two

Season Three

24

When you think it's over, it starts again.

25

In January 2016, Osterholm returned and started again. 'How scared should you be about Zika?', he asked in the *New York Times* (Osterholm 2016). According to the expert,

> every time there is a major infectious disease outbreak that scares us . . . government leaders, the public and the news media demand explanations, guidance and predictions, and often express indignation that not enough was done to prevent it. Today everyone is asking about Zika: How did this crisis happen, and what do we need to do to make it go away? We immediately forget about the outbreak that came before it, and don't plan for the ones we know are on the horizon.

Rather than responding to the latest and getting caught up in the now, scientists, journalists, and officials should prepare for the next.

> Instead of devoting ourselves to a comprehensive plan to combat microbial threats, we scramble to respond to the latest one in the headlines. There are lessons from previous infectious disease outbreaks that could and should have left us much better prepared than we are.

So what is next? Next is a 'planet-wide catastrophe caused by influenza', declared Osterholm. For the public health professional, a pandemic of influenza was (again) imminent. People must pay attention now, so that they will be prepared when it happens. The crisis was 'largely predictable and we can do much in advance to lessen the effects and diminish the spread'. Boldly claiming to 'already know which pandemics are on the horizon', Osterholm continued to palimpsest the now with the next, creating a series of substitutions, where each episode seemed to be somehow new despite its repetitiveness. Turning pandemic influenza into a serial figure that was bound to return, again and again, the public health professional created the conditions of possibility for the figure of the expert itself to appear as a serial figure, always available for another publication, another communication, perpetually going on beginning again, regularly.

26

At its root, the world of preparedness entails a political form attuned to economies of mass production. It thrives on serial figures that are proliferating in technomediated milieus. Today, the next pandemic has become a serial figure. Such figures are 'never quite exhausted by a single, definitive instantiation but always at least potentially available for yet another serial iteration'. Serial figures appear in ever-shifting shapes. They travel across space, but they never evolve in time. They branch off in different directions, but they never grow, age, or die. Nothing changes, essentially, and there is no significant development from one episode to the next, save for what is needed to capture the imagination of those who have grown weary of the last episode (Hagedorn 1995). Each repetition amounts to a renewal. With each new episode, serial figures are granted the privilege of a new beginning.

The pleasure that serial figures offer is in the movement and the variation; such movement and variation draws attention; it is irresistible and inexhaustible. What will happen *this* time? What will happen *next* time?

27

The world of preparedness is a world where pandemics are perceived as presumably inevitable events that will happen. These events are inexhaustible; they will keep perpetually going on and beginning again, regularly. Preparedness is based on the normative assumption that we have no choice but to recognise the reality of the presumably inevitable: It's not if, but when. Deprived of any historical dimension that would introduce a sense of radical alterity, pandemics 'can only come from eternity: since the beginning of time' (Barthes 1957). They transcend their instantiation, are given the 'simplicity of essences' and take on the quality of myth, in Barthes' sense:

> Myth does not deny things, on the contrary, its function is to talk about them; simply, it purifies them, it makes them innocent, it gives them a natural and eternal justification, it gives them a clarity which is not that of an explanation but that of a statement of fact.

28

In March 2017, Osterholm was back in the news, proliferating across media channels. Co-authored with Mark Olshaker, the public health professional published a book titled *Deadliest Enemy: Our War Against Killer Germs* (Osterholm 2017). Continuing his mission, Osterholm emphasised that 'infectious disease is the deadliest enemy faced by all of humankind'. The book was another attempt at serialising the author and his message. But to make the message new, entertain the public, and sell the book it had to outbid itself through multiplication, intensification, and exaggeration. To draw attention to itself, the publication had to tell stories that were somehow new despite their repetitiveness. Was *Deadliest Enemy* a response to the threat of infectious disease? Or was it response to the discursive problematic of mass media communication?

29

The logic of seriality is one of sedimentation and proliferation, a logic of space attuned to the age of global capitalism where capital, as a form of investment in the future, is always in pursuit of the next.[12] The notion of the next is a response to the 'experience of novelty and change in a capitalist culture in which change is paradoxically constant and novelty permanent' (Ngai 2008). The notion of the next embodies the 'capitalist oxymoron of serial novelty'. Ruth Mayer points out that the '*temporal* logic of narrative seriality needs to be complemented with the *spatial* logic of spread. Serial narratives reach out, take over, invade and impose' (Mayer 2013).

What, then, does it mean to be next to what's next? The persistent demand to consider what's next reflects a modern culture of mass production founded not simply on serialisation, but on the serialisation of serialisation. It has established mass media for the serial proliferation of information, prompting people to expect a sequel. Today, we are used to exploring all sorts of scenarios and find all kinds of pleasures in variations of the same. We enjoy the 'seriality of the series, not so much for the return of the same thing . . . but for the strategy of the variations . . . the way in which the same story is worked over to appear to be different' (Eco 1991). Serial figures come with the promise of making repetition a moment of renewal. They transform the future into a series of provisional ends that can be survived (Weber 2017). These provisional ends come with the promise that life will continue.

What, then, is the next, structurally speaking? Like the event of death that is always impending yet always exceeding, the experience of the living subject, whose very life opens only against the horizon of death, so the next unfolds and reinvents itself by virtue of a constitutive reiterative openness that never brings rest to the now.[13]

30

And so with this chapter: It ends here, but it can also move to the next, and begin again, regularly.

Acknowledgements

My thanks to Maria José de Abreu, Orkideh Behrouzan, James Faubion, and Ann H. Kelly for comments and suggestions. I would also like to thank Raad Fadaak and the organisers of the Fantasy/Fear conference at McGill University, where this chapter was presented as a Keynote Lecture. A revised version was delivered at the Techniques, Technologies, and Materialities of Epidemic Control conference of the 'Visual Representations of the Third Plague Pandemic' project at the University of Cambridge. I would like to thank Branwyn Poleykett and Christos Lynteris for the invitation to present this chapter at the meeting. I am also very grateful for all the suggestions I received from conference organisers and participants.

Notes

* A previous version of this chapter has been published in the journal Medicine, Anthropology, Theory (2018). CC BY 4.0
1 As Wolfgang Ernst points out, 'According to Luhmann, information only happens in the unexpected – namely, as the opposite of the redundant or predictable. In this way, the unexpected corresponds with the disturbance that is television proper; the paradoxical structure of the medium demands extraordinary events that can only appear within the ever same schematics; live broadcast would then be the condition of possibility of disrupting an otherwise imperturbably streaming flow'. Ernst, Wolfgang 'Between real time and memory on demand. Reflections on/of television', *The South Atlantic Quarterly* 101 (3) (2002), 625–636, p. 628.
2 To some extent, the content is irrelevant. The persons, places, and events mentioned in articles change, but the story remains the same. Each article about the next pandemic says the same thing. And yet, each article creates a sense of newness. That is why this essay is not interested in the content as such. I present some of the content, but only to show how it helps renew the form.
3 For the idea of the immune system as a search engine of difference, see Napier, A. David 'Nonself help. How immunology might reframe the Enlightenment', *Cultural Anthropology* 27 (1) (2012), 122–137. In 'A new sociobiology. Immunity, alterity, and the social repertoire', *Cambridge Anthropology* 31 (2) (2013), 20–43, Napier argues for a view of the virus as information. See as well Napier's earlier work, *The Age of Immunology: Conceiving a Future in an Alienated World* (Chicago, IL: The University of Chicago Press, 2003).
4 For an account of 'epidemic intelligence', see Caduff, Carlo, 'Sick weather ahead. On data-mining, crowd-sourcing and white noise', *Cambridge Anthropology* 32 (1) (2014), 32–46.
5 To understand why something repetitive can nevertheless appear as new each time, one needs to understand the role of the word 'next' in the trope of 'the next pandemic'. Hence the focus in this piece on the word 'next'. The next is a form without content (it can refer to anything). It is a propulsion, a drive, an orientation.
6 For a more detailed discussion of pandemic influenza concerns among experts, see *The Pandemic Perhaps: Dramatic Events in a Public Culture of Danger* (Berkeley, CA: The University of California Press, 2015).
7 Brown, Debra and David Orange Alert. *Learning from Stories and Reflections of September 11* (Victoria: Trafford Publishing, 2004), p. 97.
8 What the lack of a larger narrative evokes is a sense of mythic time, a time in which an endless series of events seems to inexorably follow one another. On mythic time, see Buck-Morss, Susan, *The Dialectics of Seeing. Walter Benjamin and the Arcades Project* (Cambridge: MIT Press, 1991). See as well Gomel, Elana, 'The Plague of Utopias.

Pestilence and the Apocalyptic Body', *Twentieth Century Literature* 46 (4) (2000), 405–433.

9 My thanks to Maria José de Abreu for her insight into the next that is always after.

10 Fiction is based on a fantasy, the fantasy of beginnings and endings. See Kermode, Frank, *The Sense of an Ending. Studies in the Theory of Fiction* (Oxford: Oxford University Press, 2000).

11 For a simliar observation, see Guyer, Jane I., 'Prophecy and the Near Future. Thoughts on Macroeconomic, Evangelical, and Punctuated Time', *American Ethnologist* 34 (3) (2007) 409–421. The evacuation of the present, to use Guyer's terms, is here analysed as a palimpsest.

12 'Anticipatory regimes, like those of capitalism, tend to work through logics of expansion, in which new territories for speculation must be continually found to keep the anticipatory logic moving'. Adams, Vincanne, Michelle Murphy, and Adele E. Clarke, 'Anticipation: Technoscience, Life, Affect, Temporality', *Subjectivity* 28 (2009), 246–265, p. 250f.

13 I am indebted to Maria José de Abreu for this formulation.

References

Adams, Vincanne, Michelle Murphy, and Adele E. Clarke 'Anticipation: Technoscience, life, affect, temporality', *Subjectivity* 28 (2009), 246–265.

Anderson, Ben 'Preemption, precaution, preparedness. Anticipatory action and future geographies', *Progress in Human Geography* 34 (6) (2010), 777–798.

Aradau, Claudia, and Rens van Munster *Politics of Catastrophe. Genealogies of the Unknown* (London: Routledge, 2011).

Barker, Kezia 'Influenza preparedness and the bureaucratic reflex. Anticipating and generating the 2009 H1N1 event', *Health and Place* 18 (4) (2012), 701–709.

Barthes, Roland *Mythologies* (Paris: Seuil, 1957).

Briggs, Charles L. Communicating biosecurity. *Medical Anthropology* 30 (1) (2011), 6–29.

Briggs, Charles L., and Daniel C. Hallin *Making Health Public: How News Coverage Is Remaking Media, Medicine, and Contemporary Life* (New York: Routledge, 2016).

Buck-Morss, Susan *The Dialectics of Seeing: Walter Benjamin and the Arcades Project* (Cambridge: MIT Press, 1991).

Caduff, Carlo 'Sick weather ahead. On data-mining, crowd-sourcing and white noise', *Cambridge Anthropology* 32 (1) (2014), 32–46. 2015 The Pandemic Perhaps. Dramatic Events in a Public Culture of Danger: University of California Press.

Doane, Mary Ann 'Information, crisis, catastrophe', In W. II. K. Chun, and T. Keenan (eds.), *New Media, Old Media: A History and Theory Reader*, pp. 251–264 (London: Routledge, 2006).

Eco, Umberto *The Limits of Interpretation* (Bloomington, IN: Indiana University Press, 1991).

Ernst, Wolfgang 'Between real time and memory on demand. Reflections on/of television', *The South Atlantic Quarterly* 101 (3) (2002), 625–636.

Gomel, Elana 'The plague of utopias. Pestilence and the apocalyptic body', *Twentieth Century Literature* 46 (4) (2000), 405–433.

Guyer, Jane I. 'Prophecy and the near future. Thoughts on macroeconomic, evangelical, and punctuated time', *American Ethnologist* 34 (3) (2007), 409–421.

Hagedorn, Roger 'Doubtless to be continued: A brief history of serial narrative', In R. C. Allen (ed.), *To be Continued: Soap Operas Around the World*, pp. 27–48 (London: Routledge, 1995).

Kermode, Frank *The Sense of an Ending: Studies in the Theory of Fiction* (Oxford: Oxford University Press, 2000).

Lakoff, Andrew 'Preparing for the next emergency', *Public Culture* 19 (2) (2007), 247–271.

Lakoff, Andrew 'The generic biothreat, or, how we became unprepared', *Cultural Anthropology* 23 (3) (2008), 399–428.

Lakoff, Andrew *Unprepared: Global Health in a Time of Emergency* (Berkeley, CA: The University of California Press, 2017).

Luhmann, Niklas *The Reality of the Mass Media* (Stanford, CA: Stanford University Press, 2000).

Masco, Joseph *The Theater of Operations: National Security Affect from the Cold War to the War on Terror* (Durham, NC: Duke University Press, 2014).

Massumi, Brian 'The future birth of the affective fact: The political ontology of threat', In M. Gregg and G. J. Seigworth (eds.), *The Affect Theory Reader*, pp. 52–70 (Durham, NC: Duke University Press, 2010).

Massumi, Brian *Ontopower: War, Powers, and the State of Perception* (Durham, NC: Duke University Press, 2015).

Mayer, Ruth 'Machinic Fu Manchu. Popular seriality and the logic of spread', *Journal of Narrative Theory* 43 (2) (2013), 186–217.

Mayer, Ruth 'Never Twice the Same': Fantomas' Early Seriality, *Modernism/Modernity* 1 (2) (2016). https://modernismmodernity.org/articles/mayer_fantomes.

Moretti, Franco *Signs Taken for Wonders: On the Sociology of Literary Forms* (London: Routledge, 1983).

Napier, A. David *The Age of Immunology: Conceiving a Future in an Alienated World* (Chicago, IL: The University of Chicago Press, 2003).

Napier, A. David 'Nonself help. How immunology might reframe the enlightenment', *Cultural Anthropology* 27 (1) (2012), 122–137.

Napier, A. David 'A new sociobiology. Immunity, alterity, and the social repertoire', *Cambridge Anthropology* 31 (2) (2013), 20–43.

Ngai, Sianne 'Merely interesting', *Critical Inquiry* 34 (4) (2008), 777–817.

Osterholm, Michael T. 'Preparing for the next pandemic', *Foreign Affairs* 84 (4) (2005), 24–37.

Osterholm, Michael T. 'Unprepared for a Pandemic', *Foreign Affairs* 86 (2) (2007), 47–57.

Osterholm, Michael T. 'What we're afraid to say about Ebola', *New York Times*, September 11, 2014.

Osterholm, Michael T. How scared should you be about Zika? *New York Times*, January 29, 2016.

Osterholm, Michael T. *Deadliest Enemy: Our War Against Killer Germs* (New York: Little, Brown and Company, 2017).

Samimian-Darash, Limor 'A pre-event configuration for biological threats. Preparedness and the constitution of biosecurity events', *American Ethnologist* 36 (3) (2009), 478–491.

Samimian-Darash, Limor 'Governing future potential biothreats. Toward an anthropology of uncertainty', *Current Anthropology* 54 (1) (2013), 1–22.

Sifferlin, Alexandra 'Airborne Ebola is extremely unlikely, expert says', *Time Magazine*, September 12, 2014.

Warner, Michael 'The mass public and the mass subject', In *Publics and Counterpublics*, pp. 159–186 (New York: Zone Books, 2002).

Weber, Samuel 'The new-old media', *Current Anthropology* 58 (15) (2017), S160–S161.

Wu, Lida Zeitlin 'The cross-section of a single moment': Bakhtin and Seriality (2016) Unpublished Manuscript.

3 What is an epidemic emergency?

Andrew Lakoff

The threat posed by a dangerous future event can be taken up in a number of different ways: as an object of probabilistic calculation, as a spectre that must be avoided through precautionary intervention, or as a potential catastrophe that cannot be evaded but can only be prepared for.[1] The approach that is taken to managing such a threat will depend as much on how it is classified as on the characteristics of the event itself. This chapter asks how a given disease outbreak comes to be constituted as an event of a certain kind: as a potential global health emergency.

In late 2015, health officials in Brazil reported the appearance and rapid spread of a mosquito-borne pathogen, the Zika virus. The spread of the virus was tentatively linked to an apparent epidemic of a rare and devastating birth defect, microcephaly, and to an upsurge in the number of cases of the neurological disorder Guillain-Barré. While Zika was not a novel virus, it had never before been associated with such severe outcomes. By February 2016, the virus had infected over a million Brazilians and several thousand cases of infant microcephaly had been reported. Infectious disease experts hypothesised that the virus had travelled with tourists to Brazil from French Polynesia two years earlier and feared that the upcoming summer Olympics in Rio would be a likely setting for further global circulation. As the virus was detected in other Latin American countries, some public health officials recommended that women of childbearing age delay pregnancy during the outbreak. The US Centers for Disease Control (CDC) issued an advisory suggesting that pregnant women avoid travel to affected areas.

Researchers from North America and Europe hurried to the region of the epidemic to investigate its characteristics. How many cases were there? Could the Zika virus be definitively linked to the cases of microcephaly? The prevention of further disease transmission would be a challenge, authorities warned. It would be difficult to extinguish the virus through control of its host because the species of mosquito that carried it thrived in crowded urban settings with poor infrastructures of water provision and drainage. And it would be at least a year before researchers could test a potential vaccine against the virus. As the North American summer approached, US health officials became increasingly concerned that the disease would spread to affect populations in southern regions of the country. In the face of mounting worries, the US Food and Drug Administration (FDA) approved experimental trials of a genetically modified mosquito in Florida, and

DOI: 10.4324/9780429461897-4

the CDC released funds to state and local health agencies to support Zika preparedness efforts.

Global health authorities also moved to intervene. On February 1, the Director-General of the World Health Organisation declared the Zika epidemic a 'public health emergency of international concern' (PHEIC). With this announcement, the organisation sought to galvanise 'a coordinated international response to minimise the threat in affected countries and reduce the risk of further international spread' (WHO 2016b). The act of classifying the situation as a global health emergency indicated both the potential for disaster and the urgency of immediate response.[2] But the official declaration of emergency also did something else: it brought the Zika virus into a technical and administrative relationship with a range of other public health threats. The category of PHEIC, according to WHO, not only encompassed infectious disease outbreaks, but could also include incidents of food contamination, toxic chemical releases, or nuclear accidents (WHO 2008). While unique in many respects, the 2014 Zika epidemic now also conformed to a class of event that had come to prominence among scientists, health authorities, and security officials over the prior decade.

The emergency declaration was a way of assimilating the specific event into a more general form, making it comprehensible and potentially manageable.[3] Such a process is by no means unique to the problem of infectious disease. More generally, the field of historical ontology asks how our taken-for-granted objects of existence – for instance the economy, the psyche, or the population – are brought into being through contingent and often-overlooked historical processes. Such entities, as philosopher Ian Hacking (2003: 11) argues, 'do not exist in any recognisable form until they are objects of scientific study'.[4] Expert knowledge does not only describe its objects of interest, it also helps to constitute them. In this case, the technical and administrative category of global health emergency is a product not only of the forms of human-ecological interaction through which new pathogens emerge but also of the scientific frameworks and governmental practices that seek to know and manage these pathogens. From this perspective, the invention of a concept such as 'emerging disease' is a significant event not because it marks the discovery of what had hitherto been unknown, but because it helps bring a new kind of entity – the epidemic emergency – into being.

Through the act of classification Zika was assimilated into a pre-existing governance framework, the International Health Regulations (IHR), which provided health authorities with guideposts for technical and administrative action. The first such action was the constitution of an Emergency Committee comprised of infectious disease experts whose task was to advise the WHO Director-General on how to manage the outbreak. The Committee's initial recommendations included enhanced surveillance for cases of microcephaly in areas of Zika transmission, precautionary measures to prevent infection, increased research into the aetiology of microcephaly, and ongoing discussions with the drug industry and regulatory agencies on vaccine development.

The declaration of a global health emergency, then, did not point to an extra-legal state of exception but was rather a technocratic classification designed to integrate the outbreak of a novel disease into a pre-existing regulatory frame-work.[5] The IHR framework envisioned a dangerous new world of potentially catastrophic outbreaks and bound its signatories to provisions for detecting and intervening in such outbreaks. However, while the regulations served as the liga-ture for the strategy the World Health Organisation called 'global public health security in the 21st century', their actual operation rested on a twentieth-century paradigm of international health in which nation-states remained the site of authority and responsibility while the WHO played a role of administrative coor-dination and technical norm-making (Biehl and Petryna 2015).[6] The ability of the framework to govern the actions of states in the name of a global space of public health security was highly constrained.

It is with the declaration of a public health emergency of international con-cern that the regulatory capacity of the IHR framework is put to the test. While the regulations provide criteria for determining whether a specific event should be considered a global health emergency, the effort to galvanise intensive global response through the official declaration of an epidemic emergency has proven politically fraught. Tensions have arisen around questions such as: which dis-eases should be prioritised as potential emergencies? What obligations do wealthy countries have to poor ones at the advent of an emergency? And, to what extent does the declaration of an emergency authorise international health officials to regulate the actions of nation-states? In April 2009, WHO made the very first such emergency declaration shortly after the appearance of a novel strain of influenza with the potential to cause a pandemic. When the pandemic strain proved milder than initially feared, the organisation faced sharp criticism from some quarters for its proactive response. Five years later, the question of when to declare a health emergency was at the centre of another controversy as the Ebola epidemic raged out of control in West Africa: in this case, WHO was widely accused of having failed to react in time to the severe threat posed by the outbreak.

With this backdrop in mind, the members of the newly constituted Emergency Committee charged with Zika response contributed a commentary in *The Lancet* early in 2016 to address the question, 'why is this situation a PHEIC?' (Heymann et al. 2016). The commentary began by listing the legal criteria that a given situa-tion must meet to be considered an official global health emergency: it must con-stitute a health risk to other countries through international spread, it must require a coordinated response because it is unexpected, serious, or unusual, and it must carry potential implications beyond the affected country that require immediate action. But this list of criteria did not quite address the question that the article posed: what exactly made the situation an emergency? The committee members noted that they had been asked how their decision to declare the Zika epidemic a global health emergency related to deliberations by a different Emergency Com-mittee two years earlier over the classification of the outbreak of Ebola in West Africa. 'The answer to us is clear', they wrote (ibid.). The 2014 Ebola epidemic had been classified as a PHEIC 'because of what science knew about the Ebola from many years of research during outbreaks in the past' (ibid.). In contrast, the current PHEIC had been declared 'because of what is not known about the current increase in reported clusters of microcephaly and other disorders, and how this might relate to concurrent Zika outbreaks' (ibid.). In the first case, the emergency declaration was a result of knowledge; in the second case, it was due to ignorance. Given this state of non-knowledge concerning Zika, the emergency declaration was a call for an intensive scientific mobilisation, in particular to understand the relation between the spread of the mosquito-borne pathogen and the upsurge in reported cases of microcephaly.

The explicit goal of the International Health Regulations – which were first established in the late nineteenth century – is to minimise the global spread of an infectious disease and at the same time to discourage countries from imposing unnecessary trade and travel restrictions in response to outbreaks. The regulations were revised in 2005 in response to a newly articulated problem: an apparent surge in the appearance of 'emerging diseases' such as hemorrhagic fevers, West Nile Virus, pandemic influenza, and extensively drug-resistant tuberculosis (XDR-TB). In the wake of the 2002 SARS outbreak, a number of health authorities argued that the existing international health regulations were insufficient to manage this new kind of threat. Emerging diseases had several features in common: they were caused either by previously unknown pathogens or by novel mutations of existing pathogens; their emergence and spread was difficult to predict or prevent; they were difficult or impossible to contain or to treat; and their appearance carried the portent of global catastrophe if not quickly contained.

Another feature shared by these diseases was the explanation of why they were emerging *now*: specialists argued that the increasingly frequent appearance of novel pathogens at the turn of the twenty-first century was the result of radical transformations in the relationship between humans and their environments. These changes included the disturbance of previously isolated ecosystems, increasing population density in urban slums, the rapid global circulation of people, the industrialisation of food and agricultural production systems, and the overuse of antibiotics in clinics and livestock facilities. More generally, according to this diagnosis intensifying modernisation processes had generated novel threats that traditional public health measures, from sanitation engineering to mass vaccination, were incapable of managing. As infectious disease specialists and public health authorities looked toward a future horizon of ever-emergent pathogenic threats they saw a fragile world characterised by interdependence and vulnerability.

If the category of emerging disease seemed self-evident by early 2016, it is important to underline its relatively recent invention. Beginning in the late 1980s and early 1990s, in the wake of the HIV/AIDS pandemic – which unsettled the mid-twentieth-century assumption that infectious disease was on the decline – a group of microbiologists and infectious disease epidemiologists argued that AIDS was a harbinger of many more, as-yet unknown diseases to come. By the time of the appearance and spread of Zika two and a half decades later, international health authorities had sketched and begun to implement a diagram for the governance of such diseases, known as 'global health security' (WHO 2007).[7] This diagram brought together a number of techniques of surveillance and response, such as: internet based disease reporting tools that transcended national systems of case reporting, regional laboratories capable of rapidly analysing biological samples, stockpiles of vaccines and antimicrobial drugs, incentives to develop new medical countermeasures, and emergency operations centres to coordinate response among disparate agencies. The diagram also included political and administrative measures such as decision tools to guide authorities in selecting which events constitute a global health emergency and injunctions against the imposition of economically damaging travel and trade restrictions.

The objective of global health security is to detect and contain the outbreak of a novel pathogen before it can spread to become a global catastrophe. But the various technical and administrative measures gathered together as part of this diagram should not be understood simply as direct responses to a growing number of emerging disease outbreaks; rather, these measures function to constitute a given situation as an emergency, one that requires an urgent and rapid collective response. In other words, it is not the inherent characteristics of a given disease outbreak but rather the classificatory schema as it combines with the techniques and politics of global health security that makes the event a candidate to become an official emergency. As a result, there is often a lack of fit between the characteristics of a disease event and the systems that are mobilised to respond to it. This is well illustrated by the international response to the early stages of the 2014 Ebola epidemic – or rather, the initial lack of such response. Crucially, for several months as the epidemic spread in West Africa the event was not officially classified as a global health emergency – and was, more broadly, ignored by the international community, with the exception of medical humanitarian organisations. The reasons for this delay remain a topic of debate, but arguably, at its early stages the outbreak did not fit international health officials' administrative criteria for the declaration of an emergency. At the time, many infectious disease specialists considered Ebola to be a highly dangerous but locally manageable disease and one that was unlikely to lead to a catastrophic and widespread epidemic.

As this dire failure of response demonstrates, global health security is better seen as a schema or a plan than as a set of effectively functioning mechanisms that can successfully manage any outbreak of emerging disease. Indeed, the rapid declaration by WHO of a global health emergency in the case of Zika can be understood at least in part as a reaction to widespread denunciation of the organisation for its slow response to the Ebola epidemic two years earlier. And in turn, the slow response to Ebola was likely related to criticism for an overly intensive response to swine flu in 2009. With each outbreak of a dangerous new pathogen, then, gaps in the putative global health security apparatus become apparent and calls for reform gain purchase. The pathos of preparedness is that it seems always to be preparing for the wrong emergency.

The failure of global health security to adequately manage the 2014 Ebola outbreak led to multiple inquiries, commission reports, and recommendations for reform, but did not put in question the strategic logic underlying the framework. Rather, critics raised the question of how to better meet the demand for preparedness in time for the next global health emergency. As an internal WHO report warned in early 2015, the frequency and magnitude of such events was increasing but 'the world is not adequately prepared to respond to the full range of emergencies with public health implications' (WHO 2015) – whether disease outbreaks, natural disasters, or violent conflict. The report concluded that WHO's response to Ebola and other recent emergencies 'lacked the speed, coordination, clear lines of decision making and dedicated funding to optimise implementation, reduce suffering and save lives' (ibid.). Given the scale and complexity of anticipated future emergencies, it advised, 'WHO must substantially strengthen and modernize its emergency management capacity' (ibid.).

According to critics of the organisation it was urgent that WHO rapidly transform its structures in order to maintain its role as the central organisation for managing global health crisis. 'The unconscionable Ebola epidemic opened a window of opportunity for fundamental reform', wrote one group of commentators, but this political window 'was rapidly closing' (Gostin et al. 2015: 2225). By the spring 2016, WHO leaders had committed 'to urgently reform the emergency work' of the organisation through the establishment of a new health emergencies programme (WHO 2016a). The new programme entailed three organisational reforms designed for the efficient and effective management of health emergencies. First, emergency preparedness and response would now be the responsibility of a single programme within WHO, with 'one budget, one set of rules and processes and one clear line of authority' (ibid.). Second, the programme 'would be designed to address all hazards', whether disease outbreaks, natural disasters, or violent conflicts (ibid.). And third, the organisation's approach to emergencies would be rationalised 'through one set of emergency management processes and performance metrics that will be standard across the organization' (ibid.).

Most significantly, the new programme would involve a transformation of the organisation's mission in preparing for and responding to emergencies. WHO would no longer be limited to its traditional role of providing technical support and normative guidance, but would 'give equal priority to developing and maintaining operational expertise' (WHO 2015). In sum, the programme was 'designed to deliver rapid, predictable and comprehensive support to countries and communities as they prepare for, face or recover from emergencies caused by any type of hazard to human health, whether disease outbreaks, natural or man-made disasters or conflicts' (WHO 2016c).

But these new capacities would require significant new sources of financial support. As the new Executive Director of the Health Emergencies Program, medical epidemiologist Peter Salama noted in an interview soon after his appointment in the summer 2016: 'for this program to be successful, we're going to have to find a sustainable model of financing, which is not just about us going every year with a begging bowl to donors and saying, "Look, here we are again, We're about to run out of money"' (Branswell 2016). The question of where ongoing support for the emergencies programme would come from soon arose in relation to the WHO response to the spread of the Zika virus in South America and beyond.

In November 2016, WHO Director-General Margaret Chan declared the end of the Zika virus emergency, following the recommendation of the Emergency

Committee. The decision to bring the official emergency to a close – nine months after it had begun – did not come because the spread of the disease had been brought under control. In fact, as the Southern hemisphere summer approached, experts anticipated that there would be an upsurge in cases in the coming months, and that the virus would continue to spread globally. As Salama put it, 'Zika is here to stay' (in McNeil 2016). So why had the emergency come to an end?

Recall that the initial WHO declaration of emergency in February 2016 was designed to stimulate an infusion of resources for scientific research on the relation between the Zika virus and the alarming number of microcephaly cases that were being reported among newborn babies in Brazil. As the Emergency Committee chairman, David Heymann, later described the situation: 'there was an urgent need to know whether there was an epidemiological link between the neurological disorders and the rapidly spreading Zika epidemic' (Maurice 2016: 449). One rationale for declaring the end of the emergency, then, was that this knowledge gap had been successfully addressed through the resulting 'explosion of scientific work' over the intervening months in areas such as epidemiology and virology. There was now, a WHO official reported, 'a consensus that Zika is the culprit' in causing the devastating birth defects (Aylward in Maurice 2016: 449). Based on the results of the scientific mobilisation, concluded Salama, '[w]e know enough about the virus to know that it will continue to spread and we know that it causes microcephaly' (WHO 2016d).

But in fact, a number of crucial scientific questions about Zika were only beginning to be addressed. For instance, the actual causal relation between the virus and neurological disorders such as microcephaly remained uncertain. Moreover, there was a lingering puzzle around the epidemic: why was the preponderance of reported microcephaly cases limited to a particular geographic region even as the virus travelled with its host to other parts of the globe?[8] Zika continued to spread, but its most alarming correlates did not seem to be spreading with it. Did this have something to do with the particular viral strain that was prevalent in Northeast Brazil? Or were there environmental co-factors that made adverse outcomes more likely? Such complex scientific questions could not be answered quickly.

Here is where the political-administrative category of emergency bumped up against its limits. Authorities understood that clarifying the relationship between the virus and associated neurological disorders and developing treatments or preventive measures against Zika would require lengthy scientific and public health investigation. The envisioned period of sustained attention extended well beyond the confined temporal structure of emergency. 'There are many things about the virus we still don't know', said Salama, 'and for that reason we'll be transforming the Zika programme from an emergency program into a medium to long-term programme of work' (WHO 2016d).

However, the organisation would need to find significant new resources in order to enact such a long-term programme. This need pointed to perhaps the most salient reason why the official period of emergency was being brought to an end. While most of the funding for the initial phase of Zika research and intervention had come from 'emergency-oriented donors', explained Salama, ongoing future support for work on the virus would have to come from a different source (ibid.). While the emergency donors 'tend to fund us for between six and twelve months', he continued, 'these research questions are clearly multi-year questions' (ibid.). It would now be necessary to engage with 'the research donors that are really going to look upon this issue as a long-term development issue', rather than one of acute and urgent response (ibid.).

In its early stages, the epidemic of Zika in South America and its connection with severe birth defects had presented the familiar spectre of a global health emergency: the disease had, it was theorised, travelled by plane from Polynesia two years earlier and it threatened to spread rapidly around the world as an infusion of tourists arrived in Brazil for the summer Olympic games. Travel warnings were issued and the international spread of the virus was tracked closely. But by the end of 2016, the virus was causing less alarm among global health officials. Outside of Northeast Brazil where the cases of microcephaly remained concentrated, Zika was beginning to resemble other endemic mosquito-borne diseases such as dengue and malaria. 'This extraordinary event is rapidly becoming, unfortunately, an ordinary event', commented Heymann (2016: 449). And it would therefore have trouble galvanising the attention and resources of the global health community.

For some observers, the WHO Emergency Committee's decision to end the Zika emergency was premature. 'Are we going to see a resurgence in Brazil, Columbia and elsewhere?' asked Anthony Fauci, director of the National Institute of Allergy and Infectious Disease (NIAID). 'If they pull back on the emergency, they'd better be able to reinstate it' (in McNeill 2016). Just a few weeks before the committee's decision, the US Congress had appropriated $152 million in emergency supplemental funding to NIAID as part of the 2017 Zika Response and Preparedness Act.[9] Others welcomed the committee's action, suggesting that the initial infusion of resources for the investigation of the Zika epidemic had come at the expense of support for important research on other pathogens.[10]

The difficulty of securing long-term funding for Zika response pointed to a broader problem: the disjuncture between the temporal structure of emergency as an administrative category on the one hand, and the actual course of disease on the other. In the case of Zika, the newly rationalised WHO Health Emergencies programme relegated the epidemic to the less urgent arena of 'development' even as the disease continued to spread and uncertainty remained about its relationship to terrifying birth defects. This mismatch between the rationality of preparedness and the experience of disease was a phenomenon that occurred with regularity. In the early 2000s, biodefense advocates presented the spectre of a smallpox attack to public officials, who recommended a programme of vaccination for millions of first responders; but the absence of measurable smallpox risk undermined the legitimacy of the vaccination programme (Rose 2008). Soon after that, the threat of a mutation of the H5N1 avian influenza virus led to massive investment in pandemic preparedness measures, which were then applied when a different – and far less severe – strain of pandemic flu arrived, leading to public recrimination and accusations of corruption (Lakoff 2015). The research on viral transmission set in motion by the demand for pandemic preparedness then spawned a new biological threat, one that could not be managed according to existing regulations (Caduff 2015). In the meantime, a disease that had initially helped to focus attention on the problem of global health security, Ebola, faded from the view of preparedness planners only to return in 2014 with calamitous effects.

These various failures or misapprehensions did not lead to the abandonment of the strategy of preparedness, but rather pointed authorities to the need for improved, better-targeted measures. Thus a US health official, speaking of the need to anticipate an avian influenza pandemic, testified in 2005: 'preparedness is a journey not a destination' (Agwunobi 2006). As a normative rationality, preparedness guides intervention in the present, with an eye toward a range of possible futures. But it is also more than that. Preparedness can be made into a measurable condition if certain elements are in place: a vision of what is to be prepared for, a method of testing, and a set of standards against which to measure one's current state of readiness. Alongside these elements, there are a number of available techniques – drawn from the history of civil defence and emergency management – that can be implemented or improved: exercises, early warning systems, stockpiles of supplies, methods for tracking an emergency as it unfolds. Once assembled together, these elements not only anticipate the possible occurrence of a dangerous future event; they provide the lens through which the event may be apprehended and the tools to manage it. However, insofar as there is no endpoint to such measures, we will continually find ourselves to be unprepared.

Notes

1 For a discussion of logics of anticipation in relation to the contemporary life sciences, see Adams et al. (2009). See also Anderson (2010).
2 As Craig Calhoun (2004: 375) writes, 'Emergency is a way of grasping problematic events, a way of imagining them that emphasizes their apparent unpredictability, abnormality and brevity, and that carries the corollary that response – intervention – is necessary'.
3 I am drawing on Alain Desrosières' definition of the act of 'coding' here: 'a conventional decision to construct an equivalence class between diverse objects, the "class" being judged more "general" than any particular object. A precondition for this is the assumption that these objects can be compared' (2007: 198).
4 As Michel Foucault (2008: 19) described this approach, 'it was a matter of showing by what conjunctions a whole set of practices – from the moment they became coordinated with a regime of truth – was able to make what does not exist (madness, disease, delinquency, sexuality, etc.), nonetheless become something, something however that continues not to exist'.
5 For an initiation into the literature on the sovereign state of exception, see Agamben (2005).
6 For lucid discussions of the rationality underlying humanitarian approaches to global health emergencies, see Fassin (2011) and Redfield (2013).
7 For a more detailed history of the assemblage of global health security, see Lakoff (2017).
8 '[T]here is a huge variability' in the incidence of complications from Zika, pointed out Michael Heymann, asking: 'is that simply because the virus has gone through the population at a different time, or is it really because there are other factors at play that

make one part of the world more likely to result in complications than another?' (WHO 2016e).

9   The bill provided a total of $1.1 billion in supplemental emergency funding to combat Zika. The support for NIAID was for 'research on the virology, natural history, and pathogenesis of the Zika virus infection and preclinical and clinical development of vaccines and other medical countermeasures for the Zika virus and other vector-borne diseases, domestically and internationally' (American Society for Microbiology 2016).

10   As one specialist in emerging viruses reported, 'a lot of people said that diseases like dengue have been a problem for years, and perhaps the money should be more equally allocated' (Hamzelou 2016).

References

109th Congress (2006), 2nd session, May 11, 2006 (statement of John O. Agwunobi). *Working through an Outbreak: Pandemic Flu Planning and Continuity of Operations: Hearing before the House Committee on Government Reform.*

Adams, Vincanne, Michelle Murphy, and Adele E. Clarke 'Anticipation: Technoscience, life, affect, temporality', *Subjectivity* 28 (2009), 246–265.

Agamben, Giorgio *State of Exception* (Chicago, IL: The University of Chicago Press, 2005).

American Society for Microbiology 'September 29, 2016 – Congress passes short-term continuing resolution and Funds Zika Response', www.asm.org/index.php/issues-we-follow/137-policy/documents/statements-and-testimony/94609-zika-cr-9-29-16

Anderson, Ben 'Preemption, precaution, preparedness: Anticipatory action and future geographies', *Progress in Human Geography* 34 (6) (2010), 777–798.

Biehl, Joao, and Adriana Petryna 'Critical global health', In Joao Biehl, and Adriana Petryna (eds.), *When People Come First: Critical Studies in Global Health* (Princeton, NJ: Princeton University Press, 2015).

Branswell, Helen 'The WHO has stumbled in its response to emergencies. Can this man get the next one right?' *Stat News* (November 15, 2016). www.statnews.com/2016/11/15/who-health-emergencies-peter-salama/

Caduff, Carlo *The Pandemic Perhaps: Dramatic Events in a Public Culture of Danger* (Berkeley, CA: The University of California Press, 2015).

Calhoun, Craig 'A world of emergencies: Fear, intervention, and the limits of cosmopolitan order', *Canadian Review of Sociology and Anthropology* 41 (4) (November 2004), 373–395.

Desrosières, Alain 'How to make things which hold together: Social science, statistics and the state', In Peter Wagner, Bjorn Wittrock, and Richard Whitley (eds.), *Discourses on Society: The Shaping of the Social Science Disciplines*, pp. 195–218 (Dordrecht: Kluwer, 2007).

Fassin, Didier *Humanitarian Reason: A Moral History of the Present* (Berkeley, CA: The University of California Press, 2011).

Foucault, Michel *The Birth of Biopolitics: Lectures at the Collège de France, 1978–1979*, ed. Michel Sennelart, translated by Graham Burchell (Basingstoke: Palgrave Macmillan, 2008 [1979]).

Gostin, Lawrence O., Mary C. DeBartolo, and Eric A. Friedman 'The international health regulations 10 years on: The governing framework for global health security', *The Lancet* 386 (10009) (2015), 2222–2226.

Hacking, Ian *Historical Ontology* (Cambridge, MA: Harvard University Press, 2003).

Hamzelou, Jessica 'Zika is no longer an emergency – it's worse than that, says WHO', *New Scientist* (November 22, 2016). www.newscientist.com/article/2113718-zika-is-no-longer-an-emergency-its-worse-than-that-says-who/

Heymann, David L., Abraham Hodgson, Amadou Alpha Sall, David O. Freedman, J. Erin Staples, Fernando Althabe, Kalpana Baruah, Ghazala Mahmud, Nyoman Kandun, Pedro F. C. Vasconcelos, Silvia Bino, and K. U. Menon 'Zika virus and microcephaly: Why is this situation a PHEIC?' *The Lancet* 387 (10020) (2016), 719–721.

Lakoff, Andrew 'Real-time biopolitics: The actuary and the sentinel in global public health', *Economy and Society* 44 (1) (2015), 40–59.

Maurice, John 'The Zika virus public health emergency: 6 Months on', *The Lancet* 388 (July 30, 2016), 449–450.

McNeil, Donald G., Jr. '"Zika is no longer a global emergency", W.H.O. Says', *New York Times* (November 19, 2016). www.nytimes.com/2016/11/19/health/who-ends-zika-global-health-emergency.html

Redfield, Peter *Life in Crisis: The Ethical Journal of Doctors Without Borders* (Berkeley, CA: The University of California Press, 2013).

Rose, Dale A. 'How did the smallpox vaccination program come about? Tracing the emergency of recent smallpox vaccination thinking', In Andrew Lakoff, and Stephen J. Collier (eds.), *Biosecurity Interventions: Global Health and Security in Question*, pp. 89–120 (New York: Columbia University Press, 2008).

World Health Organization (WHO) *The World Health Report 2007: A Safer Future: Global Public Health Security in the 21st Century* (Geneva: World Health Organization, 2007).

World Health Organization (WHO) *WHO Guidance for the Use of Annex 2 of the International Health Regulations (2005)*, WHO/HSE/IHR/2010.4 (Geneva: World Health Organization, 2008).

World Health Organization (WHO) 'Ensuring WHO's capacity to prepare for and respond to future large-scale and sustained outbreaks and emergencies', EB136/49. World Health Organization (January 9, 2015). http://apps.who.int/iris/handle/10665/251731

World Health Organization (WHO) 'Progress report on the development of the WHO health emergencies program (March 30, 2016) [2016a]. https://extranet.who.int/emt/article/progress-report-development-who-health-emergencies-programme-30-march-2016

World Health Organization (WHO) 'WHO Director-General summarizes the outcome of the emergency committee regarding clusters of microcephaly and Guillain-Barré Syndrome' (February 1, 2016) [2016b]. www.who.int/mediacentre/news/statements/2016/emergency-committee-zika-microcephaly/en

World Health Organization (WHO) 'WHO announces head of new Health Emergencies Programme' (June 28, 2016) [2016c]. www.who.int/news-room/detail/28-06-2016-who-announces-head-of-new-health-emergencies-programme

World Health Organization (WHO) *PIP review group transcript* (November 22, 2016) [2016d]. http://who.int/mediacentre/multimedia/Zika-virus-update-presser-22NOV2016.pdf?ua=1

World Health Organization (WHO) 'Who Rush Zika 4th emergency committee presser' (September 2, 2016) [2016e]. www.who.int/mediacentre/ec-transcript-1-september-2016.pdf

4 Migrant birds or migrant labour?

Money, mobility, and the emergence of poultry epidemics in Vietnam

Natalie Porter

Introduction

Loc's house was situated along the main path transecting Betel Nut village.[1] From the outside the property was unassuming, falling into the architectural conventions of northern Vietnamese farming communities. A wrought-iron gate and small courtyard set the house back from the packed-dirt path, which led villagers away from their modest homes and toward the rice paddies and legume crops surrounding the commune. From the inside, however, Loc's property bore marks of distinction. Scaffolding stood to the right of an ageing, two-room edifice, poised to build up from a newly laid foundation. Stacks of glossy ceramic tiles were tucked in a corner, gathering dust as they waited to be set down. On the other end of the courtyard stood a flashy new Honda Vision, its black and yellow paint job demanding attention.

Loc was a newcomer to this neighbourhood. Until recently, the property belonged to a family friend named Tho. A seasoned chicken farmer, Tho had slowly expanded his farm from a few dozen to 600 birds and made a substantial enough profit to take an early retirement in the neighbouring town. Tho's move coincided with Loc's return to the village from the island of Crete, where he had worked for four years as a migrant labourer. Using the money he earned abroad, Loc planned to take over the farm and build a new, *mo den* house.

With this purchase, Loc became the sole proprietor of the largest chicken farm in a commune known for its poultry production, and he soon found himself in over his head. His closest relatives were finishing out their own labour contracts abroad, and with most of his funds already tied up in the property and construction works, he had not yet employed regular help. To make matters worse, Loc was new to chicken production. He knew what feed to give and which vaccines to administer, but while he had the funds to instil hygiene measures, he was not attuned to the myriad microbial pathways that threatened the health of his stock. Within just a few weeks, the chicken farm lay fallow, all signs of life eviscerated by an outbreak of avian cholera.

Loc is one of many transnational labour migrants – export labourers – from northern Vietnam who return to their rural villages flush with cash and entrepreneurial visions. Eager to capitalise on their earnings, these villagers follow the

DOI: 10.4324/9780429461897-5

encouragement of the Vietnamese state, and often invest in agricultural operations. Chicken is a particularly popular investment, as this livestock commodity traditionally requires minimal inputs, grows quickly, and sells at steady prices. But in Vietnam's transitioning economy where livestock production is intensifying to meet changing consumption patterns and state development schemes, what was once seen as a commonplace livelihood strategy has become much more complex and dangerous (Vu 2009). Loc learned this lesson the hard way.

What do the experiences of migrants like Loc reveal about the mechanisms that drive epidemic emergence and spread in rural Vietnam, a region at the centre of outbreaks of avian flu and other troubling livestock infections? In this chapter, I draw on research among export labour migrants from Bac Giang province in rural northern Vietnam in order ask new questions about how transnational mobilities create the conditions for disease outbreaks at home. Sharing stories of transnational migration and return, I trace how the infusion of foreign earned incomes in rural economies alters poultry production patterns in ways that engender new opportunities as well as new disease vulnerabilities for human and nonhuman animals. These stories, I suggest, trouble existing narratives about epidemics and the economies in which they emerge. Namely, they upset accounts of globalisation and epidemics that locate infectious agents on mobile bodies and commodities. They also complicate narratives that link epidemic outbreaks to changing income and consumption patterns in cities. Most importantly, these stories expand anthropological understandings of livestock epidemics by attending to the complex aspirations, capacities, and investments of increasingly mobile, and increasingly wealthy, rural populations.

Labour migration, rural Vietnam

Asia has long been considered the 'epicenter' of emerging animal epidemics, particularly those that threaten to spill over to human populations (Shortridge and Stuart-Harris 1982). With some of the densest chicken populations in Vietnam, Bac Giang province has suffered substantial losses of life and livelihoods from outbreaks of poultry epidemics. These include enzootic infections that affect only birds, such as avian pox, chicken cholera, Gumboro, and Marek disease, as well as zoonotic infections that can pass between birds and humans, such as fowl typhoid, campylobacteriosis, Newcastle disease, and avian influenza.

In Vietnam and much of Asia, the emergence and re-emergence of these intra and interspecies infections are often understood in an economic frame that links disease outbreaks to the growth of poultry markets (Agrifood Consulting International 2007).[2] Decades-long economic growth and development across much of the continent has prompted the expansion and intensification of livestock production to meet growing consumer demand for meat (Delgado et al. 2001; Delgado and Narrod 2002). The increase in poultry populations, in turn, brings humans and other animals into closer and more frequent contact – in hatcheries, farms, slaughterhouses, and markets (Sayeed et al. 2017; Fearnley 2013; Porter 2013). New feed and pharmaceutical inputs are engendering faster-growing, higher yield poultry varieties, while simultaneously exposing flocks to novel health risks such as antimicrobial resistance (Allen and Lavau 2014). Biosafety and security measures, in turn, struggle to keep up with the health risks that accompany scaled-up commodity chains (Porter 2012; Keck 2014; Hinchliffe et al. 2008).

Further, as more and more people pursue opportunities for education and employment in cities, poultry are travelling further and further distances from farm to table, often via unsanctioned and bio-*in*secure pathways. Rural-to-urban migration has been steadily rising in Asia for nearly three decades (Dang 1999; Djamba 1999; International Organization for Migration 2003). Both humans and animals have adjusted to rising incomes and meat consumption in urban Asia, establishing a value chain along which poultry and producers move from country to city at unprecedented rates (Taylor et al. 2007). Between 1998 and 2003, for instance, poultry consumption in Ho Chi Minh City increased over one hundred percent (Hong Hanh et al. 2007). Such movements, in turn, have opened up new disease pathways where money and microbes flow in equal measure.

But these internal rural to urban movements are just part of the story of livestock epidemics in Asia. Mobility in Asia does not occur along a singular path from country to city. In Vietnam and elsewhere, rural dwellers have long set their sights further afield, and increasingly pursue short-term labour contracts abroad. Overall economic growth and the integration of Asian markets into global economies has accelerated short-term transnational labour migration, as young people seek employment in manufacturing and service industries in middle and high income countries (International Organization for Migration 2003). Notably, these migrants do not come from the elite segments of society; nor do they seek permanent resettlement. With low levels of education and a limited skill-set, young men and women from rural areas are looking for short-term, high-wage job opportunities. These migrants are what Ivan Small calls 'export laborers', individuals who literally export their bodies and return money, their absence the necessary condition for the capital flows they return (2012a: 234).

In Bac Giang province in the northern Red River Delta, such out-migrations were the norm. Virtually every family I met had at least one member (usually three or four) fulfilling a one to two-year work contract abroad, mostly in Korea, Greece, Taiwan, and Malaysia where local brokers had connections. Oftentimes, individuals would fulfil one contract, return to the village for a few years to have a baby, build a house, and/or start a business, and then migrate out again for another contract, sometimes in the same country and sometimes elsewhere. Most migrants I met saw their absence as temporary, though perhaps cyclical; export labour was a way to support growing families and begin new business ventures when they returned home to the village.

Importantly, these labour migrations were family affairs through and through, and there was an expectation that the gains from such an endeavour would be remitted and redistributed at home and within the kin network. This was in part because the costs of out-migration are substantial. In his ethnographic study of transnational migration and return, Ivan Small (2012a) documents a series of case studies in which export labourers from Vietnam pay anywhere from $3,000 to

$12,000 to obtain labour contracts in the Middle East, Europe, and elsewhere. Given these circumstances, extended families make collective decisions about who to send abroad and how much different members would contribute to the process. Families that invested in the migrant were compensated in a variety of ways, including monetary remittances, gifts of land and labour from the migrant's closest relatives. In addition, return migrants often contributed funds to send another family member abroad, displacing absence and perpetuating the forms of reciprocity that animate the system.[3]

Such mobilities have determining effects on the composition and dynamics of rural livestock economies. To date, however, anthropological research on Vietnamese labour migration has had little to say about epidemics. Recent studies in this field have examined idiosyncratic state policies toward these labourers and their everyday experiences with changing global and national regimes of migration and mobility (Small 2012a). Other works have examined how migrants imagine their identities and their relation to both the Vietnamese 'homeland' and emergent, transnational regimes of capitalist accumulation (Taylor 2000; Pfau and Giang 2009). Of particular relevance here is work that examines how labour remittances both maintain and strain social networks at home (Small 2012b; Thomas 1999).

I offer a slightly different view onto transnational labour migration, one that focuses on its epidemic effects. In what follows, I show how the process of sending villagers abroad reorganises family wealth and hierarchies and creates new and enduring obligations among relatives. I further show how income from migration infuses new funds into families and villages, thereby creating opportunities for pursuing new business ventures, including chicken production. These processes of migration, return, and reinvestment, in turn, rearrange labour arrangements in agricultural economies as families contend with more money and fewer workers. Migrants and their families navigate these changing conditions in diverse ways, and with varying degrees of success. In so doing, they foster new and unexpected disease pathways, and paint a complex picture of the diverse and shifting values, capabilities, and aspirations of rural dwellers in Vietnam's transitioning economy. The following stories of migration and return thus illustrate the determining role that transnational labour migration plays in the emergence and spread of epidemics in livestock economies.

Two stories of migration and return

Fowl, family, and fragility

There are many single parents in Betel Nut and Placid Pond villages – young fathers with wives working in light manufacturing in Crete, or in Korean cosmetic factories; young mothers with husbands labouring on construction projects in Japan, or on agricultural development works in Malaysia. Some children find themselves without either parent at home, being cared for by aunts, uncles, grandparents, and even great-grandparents.

The family I lived with in Placid Pond village included all of the preceding configurations, each contributing in some part to the development and success of their chicken farm. In 2010, I had settled at the home of Tri, his wife, Thuy, and their teenage daughter. Tri's father, Duc, owned the largest egg hatchery in the commune and was known to be the most experienced and knowledgeable chicken producer in area. Many of Tri's relatives had been involved in chicken farming their whole lives, and after Thuy married into the family several of her relatives took up the livelihood practice as well.

Thuy herself had been a temporary labour migrant, having worked for five years as an *au pair* in Taiwan. When she returned to Placid Pond, she and Tri invested her earnings in their laying hen farm. Such ventures are actively encouraged by the Vietnamese state and its Internal Organization for Labor Migration, which stated in 2008:

> After some years of working abroad, when their labor contracts end, the workers return home, and they will be encouraged to use their capital for investment and production. This plays an important role in creating jobs and reducing unemployment, especially in far distant and remote rural areas.
>
> (quoted in Small 2012a: 240)

As Thuy and Tri's flock outgrew their small backyard coop, they enrolled help on both sides of the family, housing hundreds of birds in the backyards of various relatives who assisted in feeding, cleaning, and veterinary care (Porter 2013). The couple housed part of their flock, 200 birds or so, in Duc's backyard, where it was tended to by Tri's parents and his younger brother, Cuong. Cuong, unemployed and known to be a layabout, was living with his parents and two sons while his wife was fulfilling a work contract in Crete. Another, smaller portion of the flock lived on a property owned by Tri's younger sister, Cam, who was working abroad along with her husband. Cam's 15-year-old twins lived on the property with Cam's mother- and father-in-law, in a new and imposing two-story house built with their parents' earnings. Tri and Thuy were entitled to keep their animals on Cam's property because they had partially funded her migration abroad. To reciprocate, Thuy and Tri babysat and fed Cam's twins several times per week. Even though they lived with the chickens, Cam's mother- and father-in-law did not invest themselves in the labour of caring for Thuy and Tri's chickens. Thuy told me this was because the couple belonged to a different patriline. Responsibility for this portion of the flock thus fell to Thuy's sister-in-law, Bich, whose husband (Thuy's brother) had begun a labour contract in Taiwan soon after they married. Occasionally, Thuy's mother and father lent a hand on the farm.

Though reticent and modest, Tri liked to tell me that he had never had a mortal disease outbreak in his flocks. The entire family, he said, took care of the birds' health. Tri's father and his paternal uncle had extensive chicken rearing experience and some formal training in veterinary medicine. Still, Tri worried constantly about infections, particularly Marek's disease and Gumboro. He would often consult his elders, as well as the latest poultry rearing manuals produced by the Department of Animal Health to keep up with the latest biosecurity measures. Tri also worried about the care his birds were receiving at their different locations. He was confident in his father's ability to monitor for infection, but he complained about his brother, Cuong's, lack of interest in any form of labour. He complained that Cuong frequently brought his drunken friends over to the house, and failed to heed his warnings about the hazards of strangers coming into contact with the chickens. The birds at Cam's house were another source of anxiety, since they were being cared for by Thuy's relatives, who had less experience with poultry farming. For her part, Thuy visited the flock at Duc's house twice daily in order to assist with feeding, cleaning, and egg collection, but her relations with Cam's mother- and father-in-law was less familiar, and she only visited their household every two or three days. Thuy did try to keep up good relations with her brother's wife, Bich, who she said was easygoing and receptive to her instructions. Thuy also implored her parents to make more frequent visits to the farm, reasoning that their age would allow for more easy relations with these distant relations.

By all accounts, the couple's business venture was a success. Yet, in their attempts to both expand and maintain the health of their flock through reciprocal, kin-based land and labour relations, Tri and Thuy were facilitating new disease pathways. In the first instance, the couple attempted to monitor all of their birds as part of the same flock even though the birds were housed in different spaces and under different environmental conditions. Technically each backyard farm constituted a distinct flock. A key tenet of farm biosecurity is that different flocks must be contained in their own spaces, distanced from one another by both space and time. By moving between flocks multiple times a day, Tri and Thuy were creating disease pathways for biological agents to spread. In the second instance, by bringing in new labourers to assist with the daily poultry production activities, the couple further exposed the animals to new biological and environmental agents, including infectious materials. The house Bich lived in had a handful of scavenging chickens that she came into contact with, and Thuy's parents had a flock of hens housed in their backyard. Transiting between these homes and Cam's house meant that they were also potentially exposing the birds to infectious agents and materials. And Tri could only imagine the kinds of animals and animal infections Cuong's friends were bringing onto the farm.

Thuy and Tri's story shows how the process of temporary migration and return opened up space for entrepreneurialism at home – not just for individuals or immediate families, but for an extended kin network bound together by the exchange of money, land, and labour. This was a fragile entrepreneurialism, however, and depended on the absence and presence of the right kinds of relatives. The earnings of family members working abroad generated new and unoccupied landholdings that farmers needed to house their growing flocks. In turn, these fowl could be tended to by lesser-employed relatives supported by the wages of spouses abroad. Such labour was often a form or compensation for ongoing investments in migration. The multifaceted exchanges that animated temporary, export labour migration thus created cascading obligations among villagers, which combined to effect a delicate balance of money, microbes, and mobility.

Farming failure

Loc's experience with fowl cholera illustrates just how fragile the balance of money, microbes, and mobilities can be in rural Vietnam. A further consideration of Loc's story illuminates the ways in which different kinds of migration histories and family dynamics engender monetary and labour arrangements that can foster vulnerabilities for both animals and humans.

Loc went to Crete in his early twenties as a temporary labourer to work on a construction project. While there he picked up several other contracts that kept him on the island for four years. One of Loc's neighbours told me that it cost more than $6000 USD to send him abroad. The money, she said, went to a broker who secured the work contract, enrolled Loc in preparatory language and culture lessons, and arranged for his plane flight and initial lodging on the island. Loc's neighbour told me that his aunt helped fund the trip and expected that, in exchange, Loc would help pay for her daughter's migration the following year. But Loc, she said, was young and irresponsible, and he spent much of his earnings on parties and frivolities. This was a common complaint about young labour migrants in the village, especially men. The neighbour added that when Loc did send money back to the village, it used to fund his wife's migration to Korea, rather than his cousin's. Loc's aunt was apparently still furious and had strained relations with his parents as a result of the slight.

When he returned to Vietnam, Loc was eager to invest his earnings. Like many other returnees to the commune, his first big purchase was a late model Honda motorbike. Loc then began searching for a place to build a new house for himself and his wife to start a family. Loc told me that he was still unsure about what kind of business he wanted to get involved in when he heard that Tho was retiring to town and putting his chicken farm up for sale. At the time, he said, it seemed everyone in the commune had a hand in the poultry business. Tri and Thuy were doing well, Anh had begun a commercial operation in the neighbouring province, and Sang and Vinh had started integrated duck, fruit, and fish operations just outside of the commune.

But unlike many of these producers, Loc's family was not invested in poultry farming and had never kept more than a handful of scavenging chickens in the backyard. Most of his relatives were involved in rice, soy, and peanut farming in the plots surrounding the commune. Loc himself knew little about chicken rearing but took heart from the fact that Tho's operation was established and successful. Tho was also willing to provide counsel to get him started and offered to advise him should he run into problems. This connection with Tho was especially important because Loc did not have much support from relatives. His parents were ageing, his wife was absent, his unmarried brother was working abroad, and he had alienated his aunt and her children. Loc's wife was an only child so he could not depend on much help from his in-laws. Still, Loc reasoned that because he was not involved in any other farming activities, he would be able to care for the birds on his own, full time. He bought the property and lived in Tho's home while beginning construction on a new, two-story house.

To start the operation, Loc bought five hundred broiler chickens, which he planned to fatten over the course of eight weeks and then sell off to Tho's market contact. A few weeks into the work, however, the birds were not fattening on schedule. They ate little, drank less, and began to hang their heads and struggle for breath. Loc brought a few fans into the coop to cool down the birds and provide some relief from the stagnant, humid air that hangs over northern Vietnam in the summer. When he noticed thick mucus oozing from the eyes and beaks of several birds he consulted with the local livestock supply vendor/pharmaceutical dealer, who told him to dissolve a number of antibiotics in their water. But the conjunctivitis continued to spread and the birds' wattles began to swell. Loc then called Tho, who told him to look for warts on their legs. There were none – he had vaccinated for avian pox. At this point some birds had died, many were lame, and all were emaciated. Finally, Loc called the commune vet. She diagnosed advanced fowl cholera and announced that it was too late for antibiotics to do much good. He had to cull the entire flock.

When I met him a few weeks after the slaughter the farm was in decontamination, empty and tented. Loc told me that he deeply regretted his decision to buy the farm, calling it a colossal waste of money. When I asked him whether he planned to start the operation anew he shook his head. His wife wanted to keep at it, but she had no experience either. Besides, all of his money was tied up in the house construction, which was now on hold. 'We've already put so much money into it [the farm], but it's so easy to lose everything'. He seemed ashamed. Loc confided that what he really wanted to do was return to Crete once his wife saved enough to fund another migration.

Loc's personal struggle illustrates the ambivalence some migrants feel about returning home. Despite a state-led campaign that exhorts migrants to seek prosperity in rural development projects, many labourers share the notion that economic opportunities lie abroad. As such, they hustle to stray further and further from home, signing both legal and illegal labour contracts to continue earning money and remitting it for extended periods. This is true in Vietnam as well as elsewhere in Asia (Parrenas 2001; Small 2012a: 256).

What tipped the balance against Loc? Several of his neighbours noted that Loc, young and prideful, had set his sights too high. He assumed that with just a bit of cash and no experience, he could inherit Tho's successes and become a leading producer. Others suggested that he was just unfortunate – cholera is common in the region.

Rather than try to pinpoint the cause of the epidemic, I want to explore the ways in which flows of money into and out of the commune during the migration process created particular kinds of vulnerability for Loc, his flock, and his family. Like Tri and Thuy, Loc had entrepreneurial aspirations; he saw value in a future of poultry farming. Like Thuy and Tri, he also had the funds and the infrastructure in place for such an endeavour. But unlike his more successful counterparts, Loc lacked the critical support of relatives. To keep their chicken farm running, Thuy and Tri enrolled the labour of underemployed members of their kin network. They also repurposed the property of income-earning, absent family members.

In exchange, they helped finance relatives' future mobilities, and helped care for relatives left behind. Loc did not share the kind of family composition that would allow him to seek help when necessary. On one hand, he did not uphold the forms of reciprocity characteristic of labour migration in the commune and therefore alienated himself from vital reciprocal relationships. On the other hand, his inability to recruit labour was also a function of a smaller family, a more limited flow of funds, and the absence of relatives he could call upon.

Tri and Thuy also benefitted greatly from decades of poultry rearing experience and the expertise of seasoned family members. Loc relied exclusively on Tho for expert counsel. Tho was not a relative; and though he was a family friend, geographical and generational distance set him apart from the younger poultry producer. Loc had mobility and money, but not the connections to labour or expertise needed to keep his birds healthy.

Rethinking migration and epidemics in transitioning economies

Mobility and money, then, create different aspirations, opportunities, and capabilities for migrants and their families. On its own, this is a rather mundane point. Much has been written about the cyclical costs and benefits of migration and return (Parreñas 2010; Yang 2005; Ong 1999; Constable 2003), and the expectations and responsibilities for migrants to contribute to their families and 'home' lands (Phong et al. 2000; Rottmann 2013). In Asia, migration has been established as an ongoing process characterised by periods of mobility and immobility, uncertainty and flux, as migrants and their money flow in multiple directions in global capitalist regimes (Malkki 1995; Ong 1999; Lindquist 2008).

What is notable about the migration experiences of rural dwellers in northern Vietnam are the ways in which such flows of people and money shift family dynamics and reorganise land and labour relations in ways that sustain, improve, and threaten rural life and livelihoods. Visible in this ethnographic context are strategies to fold livestock into ongoing migration processes and the familial obligations that shape it. Such strategies create new economic opportunities but also entail substantial risks, depending on the webs of obligation and exchange in which they are woven. As villagers reorganise land and labour to accommodate growing stocks, they create new disease ecologies, which can be mitigated through the right combination of vigilance, cooperation, expertise, and luck. Chickens, then, are simultaneously the outcome of and catalysts for human mobilities; they embody the aspirations and opportunities of up-and-coming rural dwellers, and their bodies (and biological states) expose their limitations and capabilities.

These stories of migration and return also shed light on an important and underemphasised facet of human mobility in Vietnam's transitioning economy – the enduring import and value of the countryside against ongoing forces of urbanisation and the evacuation of state-subsidised household agriculture (Scott et al. 2004; Nguyen 2004). In Vietnam, and Asia more broadly, migration is often understood as one facet of broader economic trends that favour urban development and redirect funds toward developing the finance, service, and commercial industries located in cities (Taylor 2007). Rural dwellers find themselves in the midst of these trends, moving in (and out) of cities to engage in an array of livelihood activities – and in many cases they are motivated by a perception that the countryside is stagnant, miserable, and without a future (Harms 2011; Harms 2016; Hoang 2015). Such rural devaluations are compounded by emerging and re-emerging livestock diseases, which have destabilised markets for rural goods and further compromised the long-term viability of agricultural economies (Porter 2012).

A somewhat different picture of migration emerges in Bac Giang, however, one in which rural dwellers attempt to mobilise toward a future at home, in the country. To be sure, such aspirations are borne of limited educational opportunities and connections in cities, state-directives, and funds, but they also reveal the ways in which individuals and families carve out new opportunities in the country against an uncertain economy. Chicken is central to this story, and indeed one of the allures of poultry production is that, at the small and medium scale, domestic fowl can be raised in families, with minimal state support or intervention. With the right combination of money and mobility, individual families can – at least in some cases – meet the demands of the industry on their own.

Stories of migration and return in Vietnam also cast new light onto understandings of epidemics. The linkages drawn in this chapter between temporary labour migration patterns and livestock disease outbreaks offer a new perspective on viral economies, one that scopes in and out, following migrants (rather than microbes) as they transit from rural villages to transnational labour markets and back again. These are not tales of jet-setting businesspersons, global health professionals, or ill-advised honeymooners wittingly or unwittingly carrying infectious biomaterials from one country to the next. Nor are they stories of virus-carrying wild birds spreading disease as their global flight paths bring them into contact with domestic poultry populations. Certainly, infections travel on bodies, and in light of pandemic threats like SARS, Ebola, and avian influenza, the scale and frequency at which humans and other animals traverse the globe have rightly gained attention. Yet, shifting focus to the dynamic local ecologies and economies in which epidemics like avian flu emerge, over and over again, reveals new links between human migration and disease spread.

Loc's and Thuy and Tri's experiences show that migrants are not just disease hosts or transmitters. They also foster epidemics rather more indirectly, by providing the conditions of possibility for intensified production and its associated pathogens. Looking for such pathogenic pathways in the globally integrated yet locally specific economies where livestock are produced, rather than on particular bodies in motion, or on particular trade, tourist, or avian migration routes, can provide a richer picture of epidemic emergence. Namely, such a mode of attention illustrates an epidemic economy in which livestock and its diseases are folded into extended and shifting family networks, whose members transit in and out of poultry production.

Return migrants' livelihood activities in also enrich narratives that link epidemic outbreaks to changing income and consumption patterns in Vietnamese cities. To be sure, the intensification of poultry production in Vietnam and much of

Asia is occurring in response to the growth of populations, incomes, and appetites in metropolitan areas. Yet migrants return to Vietnamese villages with a variety of options. Bac Giang province is a dynamic area with a burgeoning manufacturing sector, growing townships with commercial opportunities, state investments in fish and fruit farming ventures, and a budding real estate market. There are historically, culturally, and economically specific reasons that migrants endeavour to develop poultry farms over their other options – whether because of family tradition, promises of large profits, or the flexibility of the production process. How rural families choose to earn and spend money earned abroad should not be understood simply as a reaction to trends occurring in cities.

These stories of migration and return therefore expose the complex aspirations, capacities, and investments of increasingly mobile, and increasingly wealthy, rural populations. Such accounts call out for a closer consideration of what compels rural dwellers to leave their villages, and then come back to start new ventures in a livestock industry that holds both promise and peril. They reveal conflicted decisions and strained relations and ad hoc working relationships that respond in equal measure to economic trends at the rural, urban, and transnational level. Most of all, these stories depict an image of a Vietnamese countryside that remains valuable and profitable; a Vietnamese countryside where poultry and their producers are inextricably entangled in multifaceted relations of reciprocity; a Vietnamese countryside where ongoing obligations to exchange in land, labour, and money spur transnational movements, animate livestock economies, and contour the conditions for disease emergence and prevention.

Notes

1 The names of all persons and villages have been changed for privacy purposes.
2 Ecological and microbiological narratives of avian epidemics complement economic narratives. Several important studies have shown how alterations in migratory bird patterns as a result of climate change, environmental degradation, and habitat loss create the conditions for avian influenza to pass from wild to domestic bird populations (Gilbert et al. 2008). Research in microbiology has traced the rise of antibiotic resistant and highly adaptive microbes in high density poultry flocks (Nhung 2017). And research by anthropologists of science trace the ways in which emerging epidemics challenge state-of-the-art virology (MacPhail 2014; Caduff 2015; Keck 2014), as well as existing disease surveillance and preparedness infrastructures (Lakoff 2008; Lakoff 2012; Elbe et al. 2014; Samimian-Darash 2009).
3 It is important to note that these movements are not always straightforward, legal, or safe. Some labourers find themselves enrolled in transnational smuggling operations, only to be arrested and abandoned by their labour brokers and the Vietnamese Department of Labor. Others face exploitative and abusive working conditions in their destination country, and many contend with mounting debts to brokers, smugglers, and legal representatives (Small 2012a).

References

Agrifood Consulting International *The Economic Impact of Highly Pathogenic Avian Influenza – Related Biosecurity Policies on the Vietnamese Poultry Sector* (Bethesda,

MD: Prepared for the United Nations Food and Agriculture Organization & the World Health Organization, 2007).

Allen, John, and Stephanie Lavau 'Just-in-time' disease', *Journal of Cultural Economy* (2014), 1–19.

Caduff, Carlo *The Pandemic Perhaps: Dramatic Events in a Public Culture of Danger* (Berkeley, CA: The University of California Press, 2015).

Constable, Nicole *Romance on a Global Stage: Pen Pals, Virtual Ethnography, and 'Mail Order' Marriages* (Berkeley, CA: The University of California Press, 2003).

Dang, Nguyen Anh 'Market reforms and internal labor migration in Vietnam', *Asian and Pacific Migration Journal* 8 (1999), 381–407.

Delgado, Christopher, and Claire Narrod *Impact of Changing Market Forces and Policies on Structural Change in the Livestock Industries of Selected Fast-Growing Developing Countries* (FAO, 2002). www.fao.org/WAIRDOCS/LEAD/X6115E/x6115e00. htm#Contents, accessed January 10, 2010.

Delgado, C. L., M. W. Rosegrant, and S. Meijer 'Livestock to 2020: The revolution continues', International Trade in Livestock Products Symposium, January 18–19, 2001, Auckland, New Zealand 14560. International Agricultural Trade Research Consortium.

Djamba, Yanyi 'Permanent and temporary migration in Vietnam during a period of economic change', *Asia-Pacific Population Journal* 14 (1999), 25–48.

Elbe, Stefan, Anne Roemer-Mahler, and Christopher Long 'Securing circulation pharmaceutically: Antiviral stockpiling and pandemic preparedness in the European Union', *Security Dialogue* 45 (5) (2014), 440–457.

Fearnley, Lyle 'The birds of Poyang Lake: Sentinels at the interface of wild and domestic', *Limn* (3) (2013). https://limn.it/articles/the-birds-of-poyang-lake-sentinels-at-the-interface-of-wild-and-domestic/

Harms, Erik *Saigon's Edge: On the Margins of Ho Chi Minh City* (Minneapolis: The University of Minnesota Press, 2011).

Harms, Erik *Luxury and Rubble: Civility and Dispossession in the New Saigon* (Berkeley, CA: The University of California Press, 2016).

Hinchliffe, Steve, Gareth Enticott, and Nick Bingham 'Biosecurity: Spaces, practices, and boundaries', *Environment and Planning A* 40 (2008), 1528–1533.

Hoang, Kimberly Kay *Dealing in Desire: Asian Ascendancy, Western Decline, and the Hidden Currencies of Global Sex Work* (Berkeley, CA: The University of California Press, 2015).

Hong Hanh, P. T. H., S. Burgos, and D. Roland-Holst *The Poultry Sector in Viet Nam: Prospects for Smallholder Producers in the Aftermath of the HPAI Crisis: Research Report. Pro- Poor Livestock Policy Initiative Research Report* (Rome: FAO, 2007).

International Organization for Migration *Labor Migration: Trends, Challenges and Policy Responses; Labor Migration in Asia* (Geneva, Switzerland: IOM, 2003).

Keck, Frédéric 'Birds as sentinels for pandemic influenza', *BioSocieties* 9 (2) (2014), 223–225.

Lakoff, Andrew 'The generic biothreat, or how we became unprepared', *Cultural Anthropology* 23 (3) (2008), 399–428.

Lakoff, Andrew 'The risks of preparedness: Mutant bird flu', *Public Culture* 24 (3 68) (2012), 457–464.

Lindquist, Johan A. *The Anxieties of Mobility: Migration and Tourism in the Indonesian Borderlands* (Honolulu: The University of Hawaii Press, 2008).

MacPhail, Theresa *The Viral Network: A Pathography of the H1N1 Influenza Pandemic: Expertise: Cultures and Technologies of Knowledge* (Ithaca: Cornell University Press, 2014).

Malkki, Liisa H. *Purity and Exile: Violence, Memory, and National Cosmology Among Hutu Refugees in Tanzania* (Chicago IL: The University Of Chicago Press, 1995).

Nguyen, Van Suu 'The Politics of land: Inequality in land access and local conflicts in the Red River Delta since decollectivization', In Philip Taylor (ed.), *Social Inequality in Vietnam and the Challenges to Reform*, pp. 270–296 (Singapore: Institute of Southeast Asian Studies, 2004).

Ong, Aihwa *Flexible Citizenship: The Cultural Logics of Transnationality*, 2nd printing, edition (Durham, NC: Duke University Press Books, 1999).

Parreñas, Rhacel Salazar *Servants of Globalization: Women, Migration, and Domestic Work* (Stanford, CA: Stanford University Press, 2001).

Parreñas, Rhacel Salazar 'Homeward bound: The circular migration of entertainers between Japan and the Philippines', *Global Networks* 10 (3) (2010), 301–323.

Pfau, Wade Donald, and Long Thanh Giang 'Determinants and impacts of international remittances on household welfare in Vietnam', *International Social Science Journal* 60 (197–198) (2009), 431–443.

Phong, Dang, Laurence Husson, and Yves Charbit 'La diaspora Vietnamienne: Retour et intégration au Vietnam', *Revue Européenne des migrations internationales* 16 (1) (2000), 183–205.

Porter, Natalie 'Risky zoographies: The limits of place in avian flu management', *Environmental Humanities* 1 (2012), 103–121.

Porter, Natalie 'Bird flu biopower: Strategies for multispecies coexistence in Việt Nam', *American Ethnologist* 40 (1) (2013), 132–148.

Rottmann, Susan 'Cultivating and contesting order', *Anthropology of the Middle East* 8 (2) (2013), 1–20.

Samimian-Darash, Limor 'A pre-event configuration for biological threats: Preparedness and the constitution of biosecurity events', *American Ethnologist* 36 (3) (2009), 478–491.

Sayeed, Md Abu, Casey Smallwood, Tasneem Imam, et al. 'Assessment of hygienic conditions of live bird markets on avian influenza in Chittagong Metro, Bangladesh', *Preventive Veterinary Medicine* 142 (2017), 7–15.

Scott, Steffanie, Thi Kim Chuyen Truong, and Philip Taylor 'Behind the numbers: Social mobility, regional dispaities, and new trajectories of development in rural Vietnam', In Philip Taylor (ed.), *Social Inequality in Vietnam and the Challenges to Reform*, pp. 90–122 (Singapore: Institute of Southeast Asian Studies, 2004).

Shortridge, K. F., and C. H. Stuart-Harris 'An influenza epicentre?' *Lancet* 2 (8302) (1982), 812–813.

Small, Ivan 'Embodied economies: Vietnamese transnational migration and return regimes', *Sojourn* 27 (2) (2012a), 234–259.

Small, Ivan 'Over there': Imaginative displacements in Vietnamese remittance gift economies', *Journal of Vietnamese Studies* 7 (3) (2012b), 157–183.

Taylor, Philip *Fragments of the Present: Searching for Modernity in Vietnam's South* (Honolulu: The University of Hawaii Press, 2000).

Taylor, Philip 'Poor policies, wealthy peasants: Alternative trajectories of rural development in vietnam', *Journal of Vietnamese Studies* 2 (2) (2007), 3–56.

Taylor, N. M., D. H. Dung, L. T. K. Lan, N. T. Thuy, and J. Rushton *Practical Use of Value Chain Mapping to Improve Efficiency of Disease Surveillance and Control: The Case of Avian Influenza in Viet Nam* (Hanoi, Vietnam: Food and Agriculture Organization, 2007).

Thomas, Mandy 'Dislocations of desire: The transnational movement of gifts within the Vietnamese Diaspora', *Anthropological Forum* 9 (2) (1999), 145–161.

Vu, Tuong 'The political economy of avian influenza response and control in Vietnam', *STEPS* (2009). Working Paper 19. https://steps-centre.org/publication/the-political-economy-of-avian-influenza-response-and-control-in-vietnam/

Yang, Dean *International Migration, Human Capital, and Entrepreneurship: Evidence from Philippine Migrants' Exchange Rate Shocks* (Washington, DC: World Bank, Development Research Group, 2005).

5 Photography, zoonosis and epistemic suspension after the end of epidemics

Christos Lynteris

In the open steppe, somewhere in the lands spanning the Northeastern frontier of Qing China and the Russian Empire, against an unending horizon, a carefully arranged stack of numbered cages basks in the sun (Figure 5.1). Pilled in rows before the mouth of an expedition tent, the two most prominent cages bear glass fronts. In one of these odd boxes, crouches a sleepy-looking, furry animal; in the other, a standing creature seems to be touching the glass with its front paws, its gaze fixed upon us. These are Siberian marmots also known as *tarbagan*. But what are they doing there? We are so accustomed to seeing photographs of guinea pigs, rats, and other experimental animals as icons of laboratory science and its achievements, that the answer seems obvious: What else, but waiting to be taken to a lab to be tested, so as to improve human health? This, however, would be to mistake the question. For *there*, in this case, does not refer to the cage, or to the steppe, but to the photograph. What are these animals doing *in this image*? What is it that they bring into effect in and through this photograph? What is the work of their photographic presence?

Positioned within a recently emergent interest in developing visual approaches in medical anthropology (Lynteris and Prince 2016), this chapter will examine the photographic corpus where this image is embedded: the photography accompanying the Chinese-Russian plague expedition to South Siberia and Mongolia in the aftermath of the devastating plague epidemic that struck Manchuria between the autumn of 1910 and the spring of 1911. The aim of the chapter is to show how the examination of photography can help us explore a crucial subject in the anthropological and historical study of epidemics: epidemiological reasoning in the aftermath of infectious disease outbreaks. Assuming no prior knowledge of the events by readers, the chapter will proceed by briefly providing the historical context of this photographic production before launching a close examination of post-plague photography. This will be shown to embody and foster a state of epistemic suspension, which often follows the closure that characterises epidemiological knowledge in the context of infectious disease outbreaks and the public health response that they necessitate.

Plague on the Chinese-Russian frontier

Up until 1911 the main bulk of research concerning plague on the Chinese-Russian northeastern frontier was conducted under the auspices of the Russian Plague

DOI: 10.4324/9780429461897-6

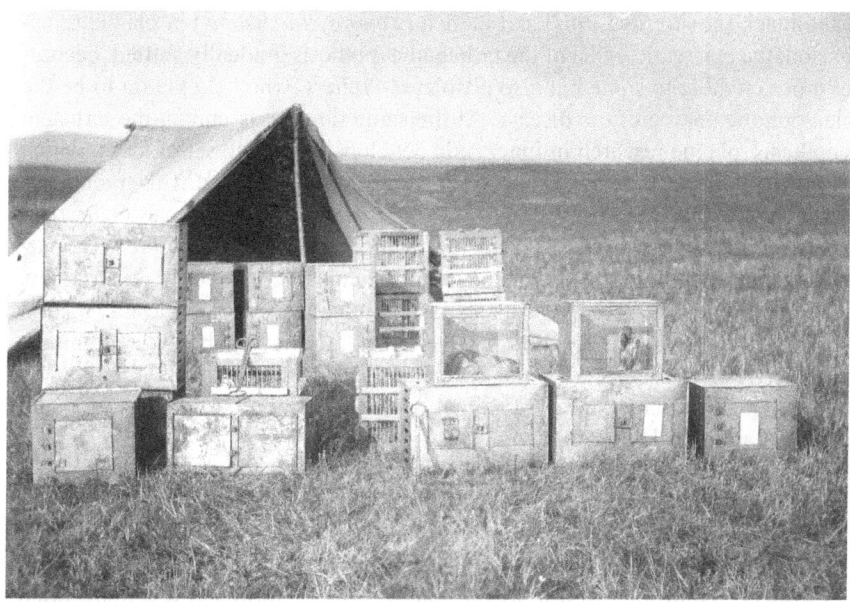

Figure 5.1 'The Animal House (Mongolia). Note the Glass Cages'
Courtesy of the University of Hong Kong Libraries

Commission, founded by Prince Oldenburg in St Petersburg in 1897 (Golikov and Sapronov 2010). Coinciding with the devastating bubonic plague outbreak in Hong Kong in 1894 and international fascination over the discovery of the bacillus (now known as *Yersinia pestis*) by the Pasteurian doctor Alexandre Yersin (1894), research on the Chinese-Russian frontier led to the first systematic scientific study of plague as a zoonotic (animal to human) disease of sylvatic (i.e. 'wild') origins. This research fostered the theory that plague was carried in the particular region of the world by marmots, which in turn served as sources of human infection. After the publication of two short reports on 'tarbagan plague' in 1895 (Beliavsky 1895; Reshetnikov 1895), plague research flourished in Transbaikalia, and to a lesser extent in Mongolia, where Russian Plague Commission experts flocked to study the disease (for detailed discussion see Lynteris 2016). As plague spread from Hong Kong across the world, forming the third plague pandemic, international scientific interest in the disease peaked. By 1910, Russian-led plague research in South Siberia, Mongolia, and Manchuria had led to dozens of scientific papers, which were systematically translated and summarised in the English, French, and German speaking medical press (ibid.).

The two pillars of this scientific production were what I have elsewhere coined the tarbagan and the native knowledge hypotheses (ibid.). The first hypothesis held that the Siberian marmot carried plague and was the source of human infection in the region. Following studies in India confirming the important role of the black rat (*Rattus rattus*) and its flea (*Xenopsylla cheopis*) in plague transmission, the epistemic value of the tarbagan hypothesis gradually shifted, becoming more credible to some but also obsolete to others, who held the rat to be the sole zoonotic source of the disease. At the same time as defending the tarbagan hypothesis, plague research in Inner Asia developed a second set of ideas, which became ever more embellished and complex as the years passed. This hypothesis supported the notion that native groups, Mongols and Buryats in particular, possessed a traditional knowledge of plague, which allowed them to identify marmots as its source (ibid.). Native hunters in particular were not only said to know plague, but also how to prevent its spread to humans. According to this theory, they could hunt marmots for their fur, meat, and fat (the targaban was an important daily resource, especially for poorer families) with impunity, as they knew how to identify a plague-infected animal by means of distanced observation and proto-hematological tests (ibid.).

The outbreak of Manchuria in 1910 had been anticipated by over fifteen years of research. And yet, those accumulated studies and insights did little to prepare the region for the extent and force of the epidemic's impact. Plague was first recorded in mid-October 1910 at the Manchurian border town of Manzhouli. The disease manifested itself in its pneumonic clinical form and was transmitted between humans in an airborne manner with no intermediate hosts or vectors.[1] Spreading fast along the rail tracks of the Chinese Eastern Railway and the South Manchurian Railway, it quickly reached to the great cities of Harbin, Mukden, and Changchun. By the time it finally waned, in April 1911, it had killed approximately 60,000 people, with a recorded mortality rate of one hundred percent. As historians of the epidemic have stressed, this catastrophic event fuelled geopolitical strife in the region (Nathan 1967; Gamsa 2006; Summers 2012). In particular, it functioned as a platform for playing out a long-standing antagonism between China and Japan in the area. Following the Russian–Japanese war of 1905, the Japanese sought to demonstrate their scientific and administrative supremacy by imposing draconian anti-plague measures by targeting the Chinese population. Applauded in the treaty-port press and emboldened by international reception of its anti-plague policy, Japan's agents in the region, spearheaded by the South Manchurian Railway's medical police, assumed control of disputed territories (Nathan 1967). Faced with such escalating challenges, the last resort of China's anti-plague leader, Dr Wu Liande, was to call for international scientific arbitration. This took the form of the First International Plague Conference, convened in Mukden (Shengzhen today) on April 3, 1911. Held only a few weeks after the sudden cessation of the outbreak, the conference was chaired by Wu and further composed by leading plague experts from eleven countries around the world.

In the course of this much-publicised meeting, Wu adopted a risky yet ultimately successful strategy.[2] Expressing his gratitude and dept to the Russians, he claimed that the source of the epidemic was not the rat, as Japanese doctors insisted, but the Siberian marmot, furthermore adding that this animal source of plague had been known to the indigenous inhabitants of Mongolia and North-western Manchuria

(Wu in Strong 1912: 19). Wu thus endorsed both the tarbagan and the native knowledge hypotheses developed by Russian plague researchers since 1894, in a move which, with the joined forces of Russia's chief delegate and plague expert of international repute, Danilo Kirilovich Zabolotny (b.1866), carried the day. By the end of the conference, the two hypotheses and their reconfirmed interdependence had become the staple of the international medical and lay press, joined together in a tight cluster of epidemiological reasoning.

The Chinese-Russian plague expedition

What is often forgotten in historical accounts of the Manchurian plague is that besides a brief visit by Wu's assistant, Dr Ch'uan Shao Ching, to Manzhouli in the winter of 1911, Chinese doctors had not had the opportunity to examine plague in the region believed to be the origin of the disease. Moreover, as Ch'uan visited Manzhouli during a period of the year when Siberian marmots are hibernating, Chinese scientists had no first-hand empirical experience of the purported zoonotic source of the disease. If Wu supported Russian claims regarding the disease originating in marmots rather than rats, this formed part of an epistemic alliance with Zabolotny in a time of biopolitical and geopolitical urgency. The latter's international prestige as a plague expert acted as a counterweight against rat-theory-proponent Kitasato Shibasaburo (b.1853) – the head of Japan's delegation to the conference, leading Japanese bacteriologist, and (as Yersin's arch-rival in the discovery of the plague bacillus in Hong Kong) a dangerous opponent for Wu (b.1879).

Medical historians and anthropologists have studied the ways in which decisions over disease aetiology, transmission pathways, and other key epidemiological traits regarding a given outbreak are influenced by social, economic, and political factors. To the extent that outbreaks function as events necessitating the rise of new conceptual frameworks and indeed of new biopolitical subjectivities (Lynteris 2014b), the challenge they pose both to scientific frameworks of understanding disease and to governmental responses to the latter more often than not results in epistemological closure. By this I mean the development and defence of a limited and largely non-reflexive set of explanations, which can form the basis for concrete, unambiguous epidemic-control intervention on the ground, and, to follow Charles Briggs and Clara Martini-Briggs' recent work, to simplified, unidirectional communication about the supposed true nature of the epidemic (2016). This has already been shown to be the case in the Manchurian plague epidemic (Lei 2011; Lynteris 2014a). What is less examined is what transpires with regard to these hastily crafted epistemological positions after the end of epidemics when the quarantines are lifted, the dead buried, the pits closed, and the journalists gone home. In a recent reflection on the 'end of disease' historian Dora Vargha (2016) stressed the importance of thinking 'after' the dramaturgical timeline of the outbreak narrative to which readers of Charles Rosenberg (1989) or Priscilla Wald (2008) are habituated: 'endings are often messier than any international, national or local governing body would care to admit, and most diseases do not map onto neat narratives. Endings hardly mean that the story is finished'. In the case of the plague, the observation that the disease tended to disappear in a given location only to reappear the following year, with a certain seasonality, was a formative part of scientific experience. In this sense, the end of an outbreak was but a temporary one. What was then the epistemic and biopolitical significance of these inter-epidemic intervals? If every 'after the end' period is also one 'before the return' of an epidemic, in which ways is this interval institutionalised and instrumental-ised both scientifically and governmentally?[3] In the case of Manchuria, where the 1910–11 outbreak was perceived to be the first of its kind, the question then arose: how could scientists, fresh from the battle against plague, take advantage of the time that remained before its potential return, so as to check and verify the conclu-sions reached at the Mukden conference?

What triggered the Chinese-Russian expedition following the Mukden confer-ence was the discovery of a plague-infected tarbagan by a protégé of Zabolotny just north of the Chinese-Russian border on June 24, 1911. Taking samples to Har-bin, Zabolotny demonstrated the preserved plague-marked organs of the animal to Wu. This discovery and news of an epizootic among marmots in Kerulen, north of the Borzya River, were crucial factors in forging an expeditionary collaboration between the two scientists.

The Russian party was led by Zabolotny, while the Chinese by Wu, who arrived in Manzhouli on July 21. After arranging for the construction of huts and a micro-biological laboratory, Wu and his assistant, Dr Chen Shipang, crossed the border for the Russian railway town of Borzya, where Zabolotny had his base. The scien-tists issued tarbagan-hunting permits to Russian hunters and offered one ruble per healthy animal and five per sick animal (Wu and the Hulun Taotai 1913: 27). Harvesting eighty marmots in total, they were perplexed by their inability to find any testing positive for plague. The expedition similarly failed to find any plague-infected marmots in either Arabulak or around Borzya itself. Thus, empty-handed, the parties broke ways on July 29. The Chinese team crossed the border back to Manzhouli, where it remained for five days, during which it investigated more marmot carcasses in the area, once again with no results. On August 4 it moved into Mongolian territory where it stayed for nine days. It first reached the twenty-family-strong Mongol 'village' of Charbada, sixty-three li southwest of Man-zhouli, on August 5; a settlement surrounded by marmot mounds. The Mongols were described as eating 'besides mutton, a good deal of Tarbagan flesh which is only half roasted before the primitive fire' (ibid.: 31). Upon Wu's enquiries, they however claimed that, 'there had never been any outbreak of disease resembling human plague in their midst. Nor could I obtain any word of disease among the Tarbagans: the country in which they had lived for many years past abounds in Tarbagans, yet they had never noticed the animals dying' (ibid.: 30).

In the meantime, trapped marmots tested negative for plague and the party moved on, along the banks of Kerulen River, where, after camping at another Mongol settlement, Wu was again unable to trace any evidence of plague among beast or human. Rich in ethnographic information regarding marmot hunting, yet empty-handed as far as plague was concerned, the Chinese party was then forced to return to Manzhouli, as the road to the plague-famous village of Abagatui was deemed too demanding for the expedition's water supplies. Wu thus reached the bustling border town on August 14, having achieved very little in terms of establishing the relation between marmots and plague.

The lack of evidence regarding the existence of plague among both tarbagan and humans (or the relation between the two) during the expedition had a decisive effect on Wu, who after a 24-month silence finally aired his scepticism in a public denouncement of the Russian hypothesis about the zoonotic origins of plague in the region. In the conclusion of an article published in October 1913 in the London-based *Journal of Hygiene*, Wu declared:

> Not only did the expeditions fail to discover a single diseased Tarbagan, but enquiries made by us directly from the hunters showed that they knew nothing of the alleged epidemic. In the experience of these hunters not only had no epidemic ever occurred among the Tarbagans but they had never even seen sick ones. In Mongolia, the Chinese expedition had similar results nor could any news be obtained of disease, past or present, from the Mongol hunters.
>
> (Ibid.: 48)

Completing his aetiological *volte-face* Wu gloated in his role as the demolisher of medical error: 'To conclude that a man whose occupation is that of a Tarbagan hunter and who takes plague has been infected from a Tarbagan is comparable to concluding that a man who sells rice and who develops plague has been infected from rice' (ibid.: 47). This pronouncement was readily adopted by the international medical community, with Russian research procuring evidence to the contrary being severely isolated and ignored over the next decade. That is, until the second Manchurian pneumonic plague epidemic in 1920–21 eventually forced Wu to once again undertake a joint Chinese-Russian (Soviet this time) expedition in 1923 and accept the tarbagan origins of the disease; a move that led him to rehabilitate the native knowledge hypothesis as an indispensable partner of the former (Lynteris 2016).

The epidemiological reasoning evident in this epistemic entanglement is a rich field for medical anthropological and historical investigation into the 'ethnographic configuration of plague' (ibid.). When we look at the photographic production accompanying the summer 1911 plague expedition, however, we are allowed a vantage point into the way in which the end of the epidemic did not directly result in a new certainty (the non-relevance of marmots, or the rejection of the tarbagan and native knowledge hypothesis) but, instead, to a return to epidemiological uncertainty. Although the expedition took place in the summer of 1911, Wu expressed his rejection of the two hypotheses that had underscored his outbreak narrative during the course of the epidemic only in 1913.[4] Though publishing delays and the intervening Revolution may certainly have played a role in this, his photographic albums also point out that Wu did not immediately shift from one kind of certainty to its exact opposite. Visual evidence thus reveals what textual ones occlude: how the end of an outbreak marks a time when epistemic frameworks, which had been developed in the course of the outbreak so as to meet the needs of a particular crisis and lead to its resolution become suspended. To understand this dialectic it is important to contrast this case of post-epidemic photography with epidemic photography per se, as this was developed and deployed in the course of the Manchurian plague outbreak.

Photographing the Manchurian plague epidemic

In the course of the 1910–11 epidemic, photography was employed extensively to cover the events unfolding in Manchuria. Hundreds of photographs were produced, the vast majority of which reflected the viewpoint and interests of different, antagonistic agents in the region. This production followed to a great extent the conventions of epidemic photography as it had been developed globally following the Hong Kong outbreak of 1894. Being the first time that the photographic lens was used to record infectious disease outbreaks in a systematic manner, the photography of the unfolding third plague pandemic brought together methods, aesthetics and norms of criminological, ethnographic, medical, war and survey photography in what we may call 'epidemic photography' (Lynteris 2016b). Numerous photographic corpuses on the outbreak survive, from American, French, Russian, Japanese, German, and Chinese sources. What is important for our discussion is the official Chinese viewpoint as encapsulated in the album produced and published by Wu Liande: *Views of Harbin, Fuchiatien, taken during the plague epidemic, December 1910March 1911* (Wu 1911). This bilingual (Chinese and English) album was presented to the delegates of the Mukden conference. Through its sixty-one of photographs, each occupying a single right-hand page, the work is unique in the way in which it engages with the epidemic in the great Manchurian city. The lens establishes a narrative that spatialises plague, rendering the disease a structural problem of working-class living space. This image rhymed with Wu's explanation of the epidemic as a result of coolie ignorance and ineptness; an aetiology that traced the outbreak to the supposedly unskilled marmot-hunting practices of migrant workers from Shandong, employed in the procurement of tarbagan fur from around Manzhouli, but also to the supposedly insanitary habits and living conditions of this class. As Wu's visual narrative unfolds, we find ourselves immersed in the dirty, dark streets of the coolie neighbourhood of Fujiadian. Then science intervenes: quarantine is imposed, contacts are isolated in immobilised train wagons, disinfection squads cleanse houses and streets, and, finally, fire is employed to torch pestilential coolie abodes. This is a narrative of order through science. The Chinese anti-plague operation is depicted as orderly and methodic – a far cry from reports of confusion, internal conflict, and popular resistance circulating about Wu's anti-plague efforts at the time (Nathan 1967). Marmots are noticeably absent. Instead the album concludes with an image of Chinese researchers examining rats in a laboratory: 'In the Laboratory: searching for infected rats'. This may appear perplexing and out of tune with Wu's hypothesis on the marmot origins of the disease and the irrelevance of rats in the outbreak. However, it is probable that this last photograph was meant to show that Chinese researchers had not neglected the potential implication of rats, but, having examined them in a scientific manner, had dismissed it as non-factual. The absence of marmots from the album is not itself surprising. On the contrary, it is exactly what should be expected, as marmots were in hibernation in the course of the human epidemic and their photographic depiction was simply impossible.

Wu's *Views of Harbin* thus provided a concise, and indeed, panoptical gaze of the epidemic: moving from the opening birds-eye-views of the afflicted city, to close-ups of coolie streets and alleys, to epidemic-control measures, and, lastly, to images of 'purification' by fire, it fostered an image of revelation and containment. This involved both what Carlos Mondragón (2015) calls a 'controlled revelation' and, I would like to argue, a 'revelation that controls' insofar as photography deployed its demonstrative faculty (Lynteris 2016b) so that the disease could be politically contained and Chinese sovereignty over Manchuria preserved in the face of Japanese challenges. By contrast, as we will now proceed to see, the albums produced by Wu Liande during the Summer 1911 plague expedition to South Siberia and Mongolia shifted attention not simply from the urban site of affliction to the rural site of origin of the disease, but also from a field of vision that fostered epistemic certainty to one that harboured epistemic doubt.

Obscuring the coolie

By contrast to *Views of Harbin* the two albums produced by Wu in the summer of 1911 were not meant for publication or distribution. We do not know the exact purpose of these albums, but they are both in form and quality very different from Wu's photographic scrapbooks currently held by the National Library of Singapore (see bibliography). The latter, whose dates of production are unknown but appear to be works-in-progress over long periods of time, contain a large number of photographs from various periods of Wu's work and career. Whereas in the Hong Kong albums each sheet carries one, centrally framed photograph, in the Singapore scrapbooks numerous, smaller format photographs are carried in each leaf, with diverse orientations and often partially overlapping. Moreover, whereas the Hong Kong albums cover a distinct time-bound event, the Singapore scrapbooks represent a mélange of photographs of events from different periods. Judging from the annotation on the margin of the photographs, in the case of the two Hong Kong albums examined here, these were used not as simple reference, but as visual objects for systematic scientific scrutiny.

The first album compiled by Wu (mis-dated 'Joint Sino-Russian Plague Research Expedition in Siberia and Mongolia 1912') concentrates on the first, joint phase of the Summer 1911 plague expedition to the Chinese-Russian frontier, in July 1911. The photographer is unknown and is nowhere identified in Wu's published or non-published works. Composed of sixteen images mounted on thick deep-purple paper, bearing hand-written annotations by Wu, the album reproduces expeditionary visual tropes that were by that time well-established in colonial photo-album practices. However, rather than simply depicting a scientific expedition, the album in fact re-enacts it in a way that institutes a visual narrative thick with hierarchies concerning skill and knowledge. These are hierarchies as much between the expeditionary force and the native subjects photographed in the field, as between the Chinese and the Russian expeditionary parties. What the album visualises is a tripartite distinction between, a) modern scientific agents (Wu's and Zabolotny's teams), b) nature-bound native subjects (Mongols and Buryats), and c) Chinese 'coolies', as a category that belongs neither to nature nor culture, but in some abominable, degenerate state of barbarism. The way this is achieved is the following.

The album opens with a photograph of the Wu Liande riding a troika with Zabolotny 'on the way to Tschintansk (Siberia)' (Figure 5.2). The photograph both brings together and separates the two plague experts. While, on the one hand, it portrays them as united in the quest for the truth of plague, in a seemingly epic journey through the vast steppes of the Chinese-Russian frontier, the way the photograph is composed accentuates a difference between the two men. Zabolotny is seated inside the horse-drawn cart, with his back turned towards the front, looking at the camera with a melancholy expression. By contrast, Wu is seated on the edge of the cart, with his feet hanging on the side, as if he were about to jump onto the grassland; his body is furthermore positioned facing the front of the cart. Zabolotny is hence depicted as old and distinguished but in a rather 'armchair' position with his back turned to the 'future' and all the discoveries it may hold. Wu, by contrast, is youthful, with beret and fashionable round shades to match, ready to set his shiny boots on the ground, explore and discover. This contrastive image between 'authority' and 'path-breaker' is further reinforced by the second

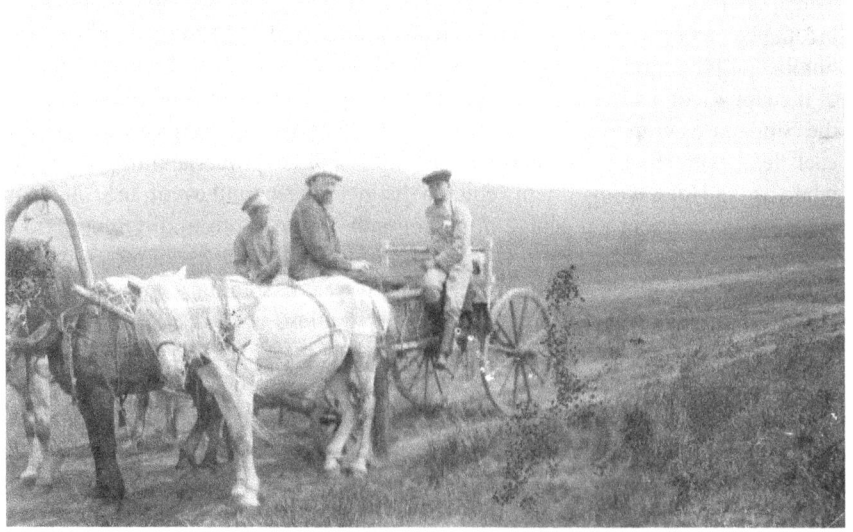

Figure 5.2 'On the way to Teshintansk (Siberia). Zabolotny and Wu July 1911
Courtesy of the University of Hong Kong Libraries

photograph of the album, featuring again the two men, this time standing on the grassland next to a 'tarbagan hole'. Here the sportive-looking Wu seems to be supporting with his arm the striped-suit-clad Zabolotny. The latter is posited further away from the marmot hole, apparently burdened by instruments he is carrying, and supporting himself on his walking stick.

Having thus established a hierarchy of knowledge between the Chinese and the Russians, the album proceeds to provide a number of ethnographic images, consisting in 'a Cossack family', a group of 'Cossacks and Buriats [sic]', the latter on horseback carrying long lasso-bearing sticks known as *uurga*, a Buryat girl on horseback and a 'Mongolian hut' with a smiling person standing at its entrance.

These images should be considered as operators of a wider imaginary of native populations as embedded in the environment they inhabited, possessing a deep knowledge of it and its features. There is little doubt that in the process of shooting these photographs, Wu and his assistants were aiming to capture nothing less than the ethnographic coordinates of plague, and in particular to provide a portrait of the people who were the supposed original savants of the epidemiology of sylvatic plague. What made this all the more important were the perceived special conditions on the steppes. Their perception as harsh, frozen, or generally wintry constituted the steppes as an environment of survival. This harsh environment was imagined not simply as key to the shape of the national or racial 'character'. More importantly, native populations were seen as necessarily more tightly enmeshed with the environment, with native 'culture' being particularly attentive to 'nature', following the dichotomy prevalent at the time. As a culture of survival, this was then a legitimate and important object of study for scientists, as it could be used as an index of underlying natural phenomena or forces, such as plague.

What brings the *plein air* vision of these photographs into focus, and comes as a visual support of the anthropological divide between native and coolie hunters, however, is the final image of the album (Figure 5.3).

This is a blurry and very dark photograph captioned 'An inn (Manchoulie)', which portrays, we may safely assume, the lodging of migrant 'coolie' marmot hunters, accused by Wu of contracting and spreading plague across Manchuria. It is hard to see anything in this image besides rough contours of wooden columns and bunk-beds, as well as an oil lamp hanging in the midst of the room. Yet perhaps it is precisely the obscurity of this photograph rather than its ability to carry or convey any identifiable data that is the intended operator here. For more than the two other images of marmot-hunting coolie inns in Manzhouli attributable to Wu (one published in the first report of the North Manchurian Plague Prevention Service (1913), the other an image in my personal possession, which was, to my knowledge, never published) this image communicates with unparalleled force an experience of darkness, crampedness, and premonition. These traits, I would like to argue, functioned antithetically to the previous fifteen photographs from the open steppes. By placing this image as the concluding photograph of the album, it could be argued that Wu created a 'surprise ending' plot reversal. This image, in its specific location and inter-relation with the proceeding photographs, seems to operate like a visual vortex of epidemiological uncertainty and doubt.

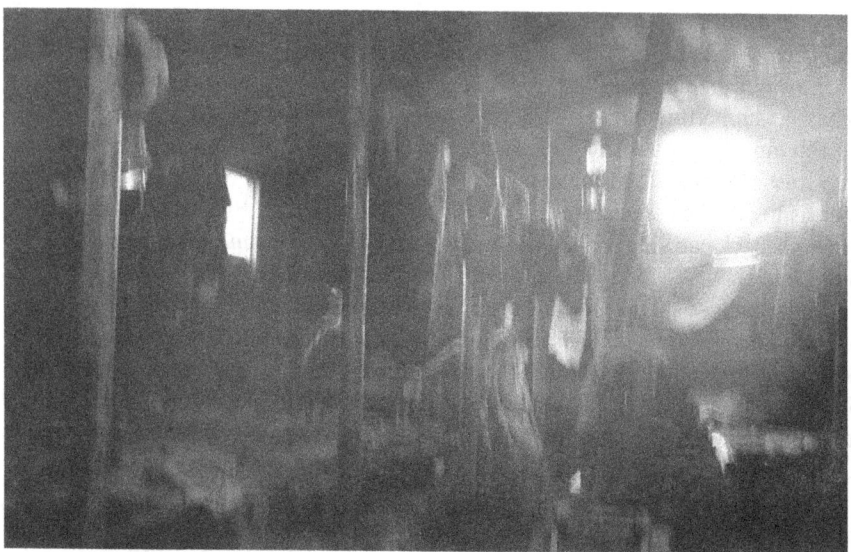

Figure 5.3 'An inn (Manchoulie)'
Courtesy of the University of Hong Kong Libraries

The darkness and blurriness of the photographs must not be here dismissed as technical errors of exposure, but following Douglas Nickel (2017) as operators of photographic indeterminacy. Where open fields and visual clarity reigned in the fifteen images preceding it, darkness, chaos, and a nauseating blurriness dominate this photograph. The viewer of the album is thus drawn back from a hitherto well-established feeling of knowledge and certainty into the unknown; from the open-horizon of the steppes, where the panoptical visual trope of the *Views of Harbin* is replicated in *plein air*, to the obscure and unintelligible interior of the migrant coolie sub-proletariat. From pan-visibility to invisibility.

Whereas initially the photographs of this album appear to have been shot as a means of visualising both the ethnographic context of plague and Chinese scientific superiority in deciphering it, in being arranged so that they lead up to the final image of the coolie inn, they assume a reverse function. Read in light of their 'surprise ending', while they do maintain the previously-mentioned Chinese-Russian hierarchy, they only do so in order for Wu to be able to disclaim the Russian plague-related hypotheses to himself and to colleagues who may have had access to this album. And, in turn, if this photographic sequence does maintain a native-coolie hierarchy it is only insofar as what is problematised is no longer the knowledge and skill involved in marmot hunting but rather the very being of the two groups: on the one hand, an originary, autochthonous being, a being-in-nature, indeed a natural being, of the natives, and on the other hand, a degenerate being, a being outside both nature and culture of the coolies. This anthropological dichotomy was already present in the native knowledge hypothesis (Lynteris 2013), but here, freed of its marmot-specific particulars, it assumes a truly ontological character. In light of this visual narrative, plague appears no longer to derive from marmots or from observable, visualisable practices or malpractices with regard to them, but instead from ignorance, as in this case embodied by the obscure and impenetrable being-in-the world known as the 'coolie'. The coolie abodes thus stand for far more than the imagined stupidity of a manual-working class – metonymically they become an icon of ignorance about plague which in turn leads to its propaga-tion; an ignorance shared by scientists who are, in this pessimistic image, groping in the dark for some answers about humanity's ancient enemy.

To fully grasp the force and meaning of this visual operation as it unfolded after the end of the epidemic, we need to look at the previously-discussed album alongside the second album resulting from the expedition. Judging from the fact that it replicates the material culture and technique of the first, we can safely assume that this was compiled simultaneously with the first. Composed of seven-teen photographs, the album focuses on the second leg of the expedition, where, having left their Russian companions, the Chinese move into Mongolia in order to continue their search of marmot plague evidence. The album opens with an evocative photograph that, as it were, bids farewell to Manzhouli through a dark, landscape vista of the steppes with the border town in the distant background. Then it proceeds by providing what we may call two action-sets of plague field investigation: exploring marmot burrows, and conducting tests on marmots in an impromptu field-lab made out of a wooden cabin and tents pitched in the grassland.

The first set of photographs does not depict the digging out of the famously deep and complex burrow of the tarbagan – what must have been a formidable operation. Indeed it is not clear when and who dug out these burrows, with a note in one of the photographs suggesting this might have been performed previous to the arrival of the expedition. The photographs concentrate on depicting the already excavated burrows with Wu's notes on the mounting paper (exactly the same as the first album) giving details on different aspects of these expansive subterranean nests. This information is mostly of topographic nature, such as their orientation, dimensions, and measurements. Besides two mainly commemora-tive photographs, which feature Wu inside a burrow surrounded by soldiers, the majority of the 'burrow exploration' images were supposed to have a scientific value as regards the study of the suspected relation between marmots and plague. Though a large part of Wu's hand-written notes on the margin of the photographs are too faded to be make sense of, the ones we can still read make clear that the scope of this series of survey images was related to the question of the persistence or attenuation of plague in the marmot burrows. Especially underlined are areas in the excavated burrows where grass or fecal matter was deposited; material believed to potentially be able to sustain plague bacilli or at least fleas carrying it. We can thus see that the question of the 'interval' discussed at the beginning of the chapter was one of pressing importance for Wu, and a key subject of his investiga-tion in the summer of 1911.[5]

The second set of photographs in this album depicts what Wu coins his 'camp laboratory'. This series begins in a commemorative mode, depicting Wu colonial-style, languishing, in pith helmet and white high-necked jacket, on a deck chair, surrounded by his Chinese guard and two lab-coated assistants, one of whom is seen staring at a glass cage containing a marmot. The open-air ambience of this image is amplified by the positioning of the camera so that it takes a slightly upward shot, creating a mis-en-scène of 'exploration' with the grasslands and hills rolling into the background. Only by magnifying the image can we actually discern that the caption ('camp laboratory in Manchoulie') should be taken at face value, as houses of the border town are faintly visible in the background.

The visual mimicry of colonial expeditions is consummated in another image of Wu, showing him taking 'afternoon tea at the lab' with his colleagues next to marmot-carrying glass cages; the first instance of these gadgets to appear in the album. The Cambridge-educated doctor is wearing his lab-coat and high, shiny leather boots, staring at the camera in a self-assured manner. Following the well-trodden colonial visual regime of 'taming the wild', to which he was certainly exposed both as a native of British Penang, and as a student at Emmanuel College, this framing of Wu as the explorer and conqueror of the steppes is equally evident in the previously mentioned marmot burrow sequence where he can be seen seated on the edge of the excavated nest clad in pith helmet and white costume with his trousers tucked into his ubiquitous leather boots as the grasslands roll in the background. At the same time, where Qing imperial imaginary had been productive of visualisations of the Northeastern steppes as a dynastic homeland, Wu's essentially European colonial gaze sought to re-configure the environment of the Chinese-Russian frontier as a landscape revealed by science. The photograph that best encapsulates this is the one titled 'Taking the Temperature of the Tarbagan'.

Here we see Wu in lab-coat taking notes as another man is taking a Siberian marmot's rectal temperature; one more individual is squatting next to them with a notepad on his lap. The photograph is composed in such way as to put the three researchers in the top right-hand quarter of the frame. What lies at the centre of the composition is a sentinel, standing to-attention, in guard of the temperature-taking operation.[6] This armed figure separates the researchers from the receding, rolling steppes, as a 'camp laboratory' tent dominates the greatest part of the composition. The juxtaposition between these three elements (researchers, sentinel, and tent) create a visual structure where it would be easy to miss what is perhaps the most important component of the photograph, and, I would like to argue, the overall subject of the album as such. This component is no other than the steppe captured between the inter-positioning of the three elements (and the 'lines', composed both by their contours and shadows) discussed previously. Rather than being a blank or a signifying backdrop of the image, the grassland is framed by this linear, almost survey grid-like, inter-position so that it is rendered a visibly controlled milieu, which is ultimately metonymised in the shape of the marmot subjected to examination.

In support of this reading comes the photograph with which I began this chapter: the oft-published image annotated by Wu as 'The Animal House, Note the

Glass Cages'. What is most striking about this image is how it visually captures the steppe. This is not done only through the expeditionary character of the photograph, by the 'extractive' ambience of the cages, or by the presence of two carefully placed pincers – instruments with which marmots were caught and subdued. The feeling of conquest, of almost packing the steppe up and taking it away for examination, is accentuated primarily by the fact that in the case of the standing marmot's cage, a faint reflection of the grassland on the glass makes it seem like the cage was see-through. The result of this *trompe-l'œil* is striking, as through it the marmot appears to be miraculously trapped within a glass cage alongside its natural environment. Marmot and steppe are by this chance effect tied together in a unique way: not simply as an animal and its habitat, but one could say as a natural continuum where plague can be examined, ascertained, and verified. This, in all probability inadvertent effect, should be considered within the history of photography's relation to chance, as recently explored by Robin Kelsey (2015: 32), who stresses that rather than compromising its scientific capacity (for its inventor, Talbot) 'the stray detail thus confirms and augments . . . the evidentiary promise of photography'. So, to return to my opening question, what is the marmot doing in this photograph, and what does it bring into effect in and through it?

A straight-forward reading, taking into consideration the album in which this image is positioned and the overall photographic production surrounding it (the two albums put together and in relation to each other), could conclude that the visual illusion of the marmot being trapped alongside the steppe in Wu's glass cage encapsulates the ability of photography to reduce not simply given hosts of the disease but the entire landscape into an experimental field for scientific examination. Seen in this manner, photography, as applied to the summer 1911 plague expedition, could be said to act so as to sustain the evidentiary promise of plague science itself, in face of Wu's failure to make any significant discovery regarding the tarbagan's relation to the disease in the region. Simply put, the particular way of framing marmots and their nests would then be said to have acted so as to assure that, having put nature under the microscope, as it were, Wu found no trace of plague among the hitherto accused marmots. In this sense, the photograph would be carrying the same function as the final, rat-examination, image of Wu's *Views of Harbin*: we have done all we could to investigate whether plague originated in this animal, and all evidence point to the fact that it did not. However, I would like to argue here, this would be to read this album from the viewpoint of the 1913 counter-thesis by Wu – that is to say with a two-years hindsight, and thus anachronistically.

Rather than closure (marmots being decided as unrelated to plague) what the photographs of the second album bring into effect is another turn in epistemic uncertainty. Both the gutted marmot burrows and the images of the marmot-investigating field-lab foster doubt regarding the relation between humans and marmots. Take the image of the glass-caged marmot: whereas on its own it could function as an image of the scientific knowledge (and control) of nature, when paired with the reflection of the steppe on the glass pane, it generates an altogether different visual effect. Not to capture, fix, or frame marmots or plague as scientifically knowable and actionable categories, nor, however, to affirm or reproduce human mastery over these animals or on 'nature' as a whole – but, rather, to situate all of the above within an aporetic visual field; a field where marmots' disease status and their role in human plague remain unstable, undecidable, and uncertain.

Conclusion

If in the realm of medical science human mastery over human-animal relations generally proceeds from human knowledge of the latter, the role of marmots in the photographic production accompanying the summer 1911 plague expedition to the Chinese-Russian frontier acts as a case where the visualisation of animals by scientists fosters a vision of epistemological suspension. Visible yet unseen, knowable but unknown, ascertainable and yet elusive, the zoonotic transmission link was not established, reproduced, or stabilised, nor, on the other hand, negated or debunked through photographic practice. Instead it was rendered irresolute, indefinite, and suspect. The vision of plague produced after the end of the epidemic, in the imagined interval before its recrudescence, undid the epistemic closure so carefully crafted in the course of the First International Plague Conference in Mukden a few months earlier without leading yet to another closure, a formulated antithesis of the original thesis. Examining the photographic archive of epidemiological work thus allows us a rare glimpse of the suspended step of epidemiological reasoning in the time after the end of epidemics – a step that, whether methodic or not, is often erased or silenced in written documents but whose study may allow for greater phenomenological clarity on the work of epidemiological judgement.

Acknowledgements

Research leading to this chapter was funded by the European Research Council under the European Union's Seventh Framework Programme (FP/2007–13)/ ERC Grant Agreement no. 336564 for the project 'Visual Representations of the Third Plague Pandemic' at the University of Cambridge and the University of St Andrews. I would like to thank the Special Collections of the Hong Kong University Library for making Wu Liande's albums available for examination. I would also like to thank the organisers and participants of the East Asia Seminar at the Faculty of Asian and Middle Eastern Studies of the University of Cambridge for their feedback on an earlier version of this work, and Dora Vargha and the participants of the 'After the End of Disease' conference at Birkberk College for stimulating an ongoing, thought-provoking discussion of historical and anthropological perspectives of post-epidemic epistemologies and biopolitics.

Notes

1 Pneumonic plague is one of the three principal clinical forms of plague in humans; it is a condition that may develop from an initial infection of the lymph nodes or directly if contracted in an airborne manner from humans, cats, or other animals.

2 The minutes of the conference would be later published, with some omissions, in Manila under the editorship of Richard Pearson Strong (1912), covering 500 pages of dense reports and discussion; the published report also contained images of marmots.

3 I have elsewhere examined how, in Hong Kong and British India, scientific focus and governmental anxiety over this interval fostered ideas about the invisibility of plague, leading to what we may call plague's crypto-topologies: situated materialities where plague could become attenuated before it was able to strike again (Lynteris 2017; Lynteris in print).

4 The fact that no diaries by Wu survive from the months immediately following the end of the epidemic makes these photographs a unique historical source. As is often the case, this is also a source riddled with problems. We do not know who took the photographs, or how many photographs were taken, with what sort of camera or film. We do not know how the photographs in the albums were selected, who mounted the albums and who used them after they were created or to what purpose. All that remains is the visual objects themselves, including a few notes taken on the paper on which the photographs were mounted, and the reproduction of some of these photos in the publications of the North Manchurian Plague Prevention Service and of Wu Liande.

5 The final three photographs of the album do not depict the expedition but are copies from *Views of Harbin*. The first two are of plague burials. They first depicts 'Coffins scattered in the open fields of Fuchiatien, Harbin, during pneumonic plague epidemic, Jan. 1911'), while the second 'Dr. Graham Aspland (C.M.S. Mission) during service on the occasion of cremation of Roman Catholic converts, Pneumonic Plague Epidemic, March, 1911, HARBIN'. The third and final photo bears no caption and depicts the torching of the first plague hospital in Harbin, which was considered by Wu to be so infected that it had to be destroyed even as the outbreak was raging. We may assume these were added later, as they do not bear the characteristic hand-written caption by Wu.

6 For the broader importance on sentinels in epidemiological thinking, see Keck (2014).

Bibliography

Unpublished sources

Extra Plague Scenes, Principally 1910–11 and 1920–21 and Cholera; Chronological Record of Anti-Plague Work in Manchuria and China 1910–1937 [National Library Board, Singapore B20062870C].

Joint Sino-Russian Plague Research Expedition in Siberia and Mongolia 1912 [Hong Kong University Library Special Collections U 614.4957 J7].

Plague and Medical Sciences, Manchuria and China, 1911, 1921 up to 1936 [National Library Board, Singapore B20062869K].

Views of Chinese plague epidemic expedition in west Manchuria, 1911 / headed by W.L.T; [Hong Kong University Library Special Collections, U 614.49518 W9].

Primary published sources

Beliavsky, M. E. 'O chumê tarbaganov: Zapiska po povodu 7 smertnuikh sluchaev ot upotrebleniya v pishchu surkov, porazhennuikh chumoyu v poselkê Soktuevskom', *Vestnik obshchestvennoĭ gigienui, sudebnoĭ i prakticheskoĭ meditsinui* 23 (2) (1895), 1–6.

Reshetnikov, A. 'O chumê tarbaganov, perenesennoĭ na lyudeĭ', *Vestnik obshchestvennoĭ gigienui, sudebnoĭ i prakticheskoĭ meditsinui* 23 (2) (1895), 6–9.

Strong, Richard P., ed. *Report of the International Plague Conference (held at Mukden in April 1911* (Manila: Bureau of Printing, 1912).

Wu, Lien-Teh *Views of Harbin, Fuchiatien, taken during the plague epidemic*, December 1910–March 1911 (Shanghai: n. p., 1911).

Wu, Lien-The, and The Hulun Taotai, 'First report of the north manchurian plague prevention service', *The Journal of Hygiene* 13 (3) (October 1913), 237–290.

Yersin, Alexandre 'La peste bubonique à Hong Kong', *Annales de l' Institut Pasteur* 8 (1894), 662–667.

Secondary published sources

Briggs, Charles L., and C. Mantini-Briggs *Tell Me Why My Children Died: Rabies, Indigenous Knowledge, and Communicative Justice* (Durham, NC: Duke University Press, 2016).

Gamsa, Mark 'The epidemic of pneumonic plague in Manchuria 1910–1911', *Past and Present* 90 (2006), 147–184.

Golikov, Yu P., and N. S. Sapronov *Popechitel' Imperatorskogo Instituta Eksperimentalnoĭ Meditsinui prints Aleksandr Petrovich Oldenburgsky* (St Petersburg: Rostok, 2010).

Keck, Frédéric 'From purgatory to sentinel: "forms/events" in the field of zoonoses', *The Cambridge Journal of Anthropology* 32 (1) (2014), 47–61.

Kelsey, Robert *Photography and the Art of Chance* (Cambridge, MA: The Belknap Press of Harvard University Press, 2015).

Lei, S. H. L. 'Sovereignty and the microscope: Constituting notifiable infectious disease and containing the Manchurian plague (1910–11)', In A. K. C. Leung, and C. Furth (eds.), *Health and Hygiene in Chinese East Asia: Policies and Publics in the Long Twentieth Century*, pp. 73–106 (Durham, NC: Duke University Press, 2011).

Lynteris, Christos 'Skilled natives, inept coolies. Marmot hunting and the great Manchurian pneumonic plague (1910–1911)', *History and Anthropology* 24 (3) (2013), 303–321.

Lynteris, Christos 'Introduction: The time of epidemics', *Cambridge Anthropology* 32 (1) (2014a), 24–31.

Lynteris, Christos 'Epidemics as events and as crises: Comparing two plague outbreaks in Manchuria (1910–11 and 1920–21)', *Cambridge Anthropology* 32 (1) (2014b), 62–76.

Lynteris, Christos *Ethnographic Plague: Configuring Disease on the Chinese-Russian Frontier* (London: Palgrave Macmillan, 2016a).

Lynteris, Christos 'The Prophetic faculty of epidemic photography: Chinese wet markets and the imagination of the next pandemic', *Visual Anthropology* 29 (2) Special Issue: Medicine, Photography and Anthropology (2016b), 118–132.

Lynteris, Christos 'A suitable soil: Plague's breeding grounds at the dawn of the third pandemic', *Medical History* 61 (3) (June 2017), 343–357.

Lynteris, Christos 'Pestis minor: The history of a contested plague pathology', *Bulletin of the History of Medicine* (in print).

Lynteris, Christos, and Ruth J. Prince 'Anthropology and medical photography: Ethnographic, critical and comparative perspectives', *Visual Anthropology* 29 (2) Special Issue: Medicine, Photography and Anthropology (2016), 101–117.

Mondragón, Carlos 'Concealment, revelation and cosmological dualism. Visibility, materiality and the spiritscape of the Torres Islands, Vanuatu', *Cahiers d'anthropologie sociale* 11 Montrer/Occulter. Visibilité et contextes rituels (2015), 38–50.

Nathan, Carl F. *Plague Prevention and Politics in Manchuria 1910–1931* (Cambridge, MA: Harvard East Asian Monographs, 1967).

Nickel, Douglas R. 'Three or four kinds of indeterminacy in the photograph', In Sabine T. Kriebel, and Andrés Mario Zervigón (eds.), *Photography and Doubt*, pp. 10–25 (London and New York: Routledge, 2017).

Rosenberg, Charles 'What is an epidemic? AIDS in historical perspective', *Daedalus* 118 (2) Living with AIDS (Spring 1989), 1–17.

Summers, William C. *The Great Manchurian Plague 1910–1911* (New Haven, CT: Yale University Press, 2012).

Vargha, Dora 'After the end of disease: Rethinking the epidemic narrative', *Somatosphere* (May 17, 2016). http://somatosphere.net/2016/05/after-the-end-of-disease-rethinking-the-epidemic-narrative.html

Wald, Priscilla *Contagious: Cultures, Carriers, and the Outbreak Narrative* (Durham, NC: Duke University Press, 2008).

6 The multispecies infrastructure of zoonosis

Genese Marie Sodikoff

Hiding in vessels of various kinds – ships, train-wagons, cars – and feeding on grain and other human food stores, rats, in modern times, carried bubonic plague around the world. By the end of the nineteenth century, maritime trade and travel had spread the pathogen to every continent, as flea-ridden, bacteria-carrying rats scurried on and off vessels at seaports (Echenberg 2002). Although rats were never plague's sole host, by 1898 they were identified as the main agents of what became known as the 'third plague pandemic', originating in Yunnan, China in the mid-nineteenth century and 'girdling the Earth' within several decades (Anonymous 1910: SM7; Simond 1898; Echenberg 2007; Little 2011; Buell 2012; Lynteris 2016; Evans 2018).

Attempts were made to control the 'vermin' on board vessels with cats. Yet the structure of ships offered deep hiding spaces that thwarted feline ratters, so fumigation eventually became the best option (Anonymous 1900: 319; Anonymous 1914: 928; Engelmann 2018; Evans 2018). 'Let no rat take passage on any ship whatsoever, and if at the port of destination any rat is found on board, the penalty which he shall suffer is death', writes a United States Public Health official in 1913 (Rucker 1913: 163). Plague-control efforts on land, unlike on ships, confronted the challenge of limitless escape routes: when people eradicated rats and fleas from one area, rats fled to new territories, where plague outbreaks eventually erupted.

While human transportation networks trafficked plague-carrying rats far and wide, underground animal-built networks have played an important role in sustaining plague outbreak cycles within regions. Scientific investigations into the burrow systems of rats, gerbils, mice, shrews, rabbits, marmots, prairie dogs, and other small animals have shed light on the plague's transmission routes, persistence, and seasonal periodicity (Thiessen and Maxwell 1979; Friggens et al. 2010; Schmid et al. 2012; Wilschut et al. 2015; Zeppelini et al. 2016). Burrow systems create zoonotic 'hotspots', landscapes in which 'the sudden, ephemeral, and material concurrences between humans, animals, non-humans, institutions, and pasts' give rise to animal-to-human contagion (Brown and Kelly 2014: 292).

In this chapter, I examine the multispecies, multi-layered 'infrastructures' that have enabled the circulation and persistence of *Yersina pestis*, the plague bacillus (see Morita 2017). I focus on Madagascar, where I have been conducting ethnographic research on recent outbreaks since 2015. Madagascar reports a third of the world's plague cases today and has grappled with the disease since its introduction

DOI: 10.4324/9780429461897-7

to the island in 1898 (Kreppel 2014). From August to November 2017, the island suffered its worst outbreak of bubonic and pneumonic plague in fifty years, with a total of 2,348 confirmed, probable, and suspected, and 202 deaths (World Health Organization 2017).

Black rats (*Rattus rattus*) and brown rats (*Rattus norvegicus*) are plague's dominant host species on the island, although other faunal species, such as domesticated rabbits and guinea pigs, have contracted the plague spontaneously, while lemurs infected with *Y. pestis* in laboratory tests during the early twentieth century have proven to be highly susceptible to the plague (Girard and Estrade 1934; Brygoo 1966: 31). Plague outbreaks in Madagascar have become more frequent and deadly over the past twenty-five years, in part as an effect of climate change. The problems of hygiene and rat control remain as salient in public health discourse today as they were at the turn of the twentieth century.

'Infrastructure' in the anthropological literature has been conceptualised as a bulwark of systems and networks that undergirds modern social life and enables the flow of resources (Star 1999; von Schnitzler 2013; Larkin 2008, 2013). By connecting up localities at diverse scales and circulating goods and information, infrastructures have been considered integral to the formation of modern subjectivities (Star 1999; Anand 2017; Larkin 2013; Kosoy and Bakker 2008; Dourish and Bell 2007). They have also been analysed as essentially human productions, including non-material networks of communication and economic activity (Simone 2004; Elyachar 2010). If instead we approach 'infrastructure' through a multispecies ethnographic lens, we see how obstructions to desirable resource flows can stem from non-human bodies and energy expenditures, as much as from unequal (human) social relations of power and privilege. Non-human life forms can taint the substance of flow, and non-human spatial formations can sometimes detrimentally impact material installations.

The goal of vanquishing plague's reservoir has eluded authorities in Madagascar, and rodent burrows may help to explain why. As systems that enable rodents to travel, reproduce, hide from predators, store food, and link up sources of food on the surface, burrows comprise a network through which *Y. pestis* circulates in animal and insect bodies, seasonally emerging to infect human populations. As structures instinctively generated by non-human species according to their body plans and energy expenditures, burrows represent what Henri Lefebvre (1991) has called a 'spatial architectonics'. Rodent architectonics in Madagascar has responded to the threats and benefits of humanity's various projects and enterprises. It has shaped the direction and velocity of plague's spread on the island, as well as its persistence (McCormick 2003; Wilschut et al. 2013). Burrow systems thus comprise an *infra*-infra-structure of plague, a substratum of 'the embedded technical backdrop of social flows and exchanges' (Chu 2014: 353; Star 1999).

Infrastructures as multispecies productions

Beyond political and economic causes of infrastructural breakdown, it often happens that installations collapse or must be redesigned due to the impacts of other creatures. In urban spaces, rodent tunnels and burrows weaken and destroy infrastructure by 'digging out the soil underneath' sidewalks and walls (Fleischer et al. 2017). Burrowed streets and sidewalks can collapse under the weight of the passersby. Beyond their physical impacts on urban environments, rodent tunnels have thwarted public health networks and systems implemented to control infectious disease outbreaks. As colonial scientists noted, sanitary cordons and quarantines meant to limit the circulation of contagious people and merchandise did little good when it came to rats (Blanchy 1995).

Paul-Louis Simond's discovery in 1898 that rodents carried the plague, and their fleas inoculated humans with tainted blood, did not immediately impact plague-control strategies (Simond et al. 1998). Nicholas Evans (2018: 24) writes that the 'rat-flea theory of plague propagation', which Simond had proposed early in the Bombay epidemic, was incrementally endorsed over the following years by 'increasing numbers of physicians in India and abroad'.

Theories about miasma, or noxious vapours emitted from soils, had given way to a bacteriological understanding of soils' role in harbouring the bacillus (Lynteris 2017b). The rat-flea theory did not supplant the infectious soil hypothesis but was in fact complementary to it as soil came to be seen as the 'breeding ground of rats' (Engelmann 2018: 368). Between 1894 and 1926, scientists had taken a keener interest in studying the terrestrial formations built by rodents, the invisible spaces of their social lives. They were especially intrigued by ethnographic data about relations between people and disease hosts that gave insights into mechanisms of plague transmission (Lynteris 2016). On this point, my own ethnographic research has investigated human-rat encounters – both those experienced by rural residents and those conjectured by scientists – in a plague zone of rural Madagascar, which I discuss in the final section of this chapter.

In contemporary times, the role of burrow systems in the cyclicity of plague outbreaks in animals and humans has emerged as an important object of scientific study. Enzootic, epizootic, and zoonotic cycles of the plague refer to bacterial thresholds in the reservoir species. As Lynteris explains:

> If 'zoonotic' signifies the moment where animal-to-human infection is actualised, 'enzootic' refers to a process during which a pathogen circulates within a given animal population without any major mortality observed. 'Epizootic', in turn, refers to phenomena of kill-offs or massive mortality events during which large numbers of the host population become infected and die. In this way, the various agents of plague (humans, domestic animals, wild animals, fleas) and their linkages are situated on three overlapping pathogenic fields, whose dynamic spatial inter-positioning plays a vital role in the hierarchical integration of the said agents into the visual field of zoonosis.
>
> (Lynteris 2017a: 472)

In their study of prairie dogs in the American West, Zeppelini et al. (2016: 3) analyse the potential roles of 'burrow cities' in harbouring plague bacteria. One hypothesis is that after sections of the burrow cities are thinned out, say after a large kill-off by plague or poison, adjacent rodent populations may move into the niche, which still may contain infectious fleas or individuals. Rodent subpopulations inhabiting various parts of these burrow cities move continuously through their interconnected crawlways, enabling the survival of the pathogen over time, regardless of large kill-offs. In their study of prairie dog burrows, Friggens et al. (2010) hypothesise that burrows act as sites of flea exchange among prairie dogs, and between prairie dogs and ground squirrels, thus playing a role in recurrent plague outbreaks.

Burrow corridors can indicate the direction of plague's spread. In their study of plague outbreak data and satellite images of great gerbil burrows in eastern Kazakhstan, Wilschut et al. (2013) found that burrow corridors do not extend over space in random fashion but are contoured by functional geographic barriers, such as lakes, rivers, and sand dunes. Using plague data from 1949 to 1995, Wilschut et al. perceived that burrow systems largely followed a North-West-South-East alignment, and that landscape features guided their construction. Gerbils forage vegetation near the openings of their burrows, so greener areas possessed a higher density of burrows. The systems stretched along the sides of dunes, rather than across them, perhaps to avoid predators. Also, gerbils tended to avoid *takirs* (lakes formed in depressions after snow melt), where the soil is clay-rich. The authors believe that the clayey soils, once settled, are difficult for gerbils to dig (Wilschut et al. 2013).

On the highly biodiverse island of Madagascar, the only endemic rodent that constructs burrows is the nocturnal Giant Jumping Rat (*Hypogeomys antimena*), which occupies dry deciduous forest on the west coast and spends its days underground (Sommer et al. 2002). Only one flea species, *Xenopsylla petteri*, infests this animal, however, and this flea is not a plague vector.

The exotic black rat, originally arboreal, also burrows. An extensive 1966 study of fleas and rat structures around the Antananarivo region was undertaken by J. M. Klein, a scientist with France's *Office de la Recherche Scientifique et Technique Outre-mer* (ORSTOM) (since renamed the *Institut de Recherche pour le Développement* (IRD)). His team was especially interested in learning more about the endemic flea, *Sinopsyllus fonquerniei*, one of two vectoring flea species in Madagascar, the other being the exotic species, *Xenopsylla cheopis*. Each occupies its distinct niche and follows a different seasonal rhythm (Klein 1966: 20; Duchemin 2003). *S. fonquerniei* lives in cooler altitudes above 800 metres and mainly infests outdoor rats, whereas *X. cheopis* mainly prefers rats found in dwellings.[1]

Within the parameters of the study site, Klein's team (including himself, a research assistant, and a manual worker) examined a total of 412 rats' burrow-nests, most of them perforating the edges of rice fields during the harvest months from March to June. About a third of the burrows discovered were dug near dry crops, mainly cassava, and about twenty percent were bored into 'ditch walls, in uncultivated mounds covered with agaves and guavas or along creeks, more or less away from crops' (Klein 1966: 7). Burrows of the common house mouse (*Mus musculus*) are also commonly found in the bunds of paddies, and can be distinguished from rat burrows by the smaller diameter of the galleries.

Klein's study, which I translate from the French, illustrates the multispecies quality of rats' burrow systems. He offers a detailed description of the architecture, contents of the nesting 'litter', and successive occupants of the rat burrow system. The burrows possess a

> simple structure and always open on a vertical wall or slope. . . . They include 1 to 3 holes, a horizontal gallery 10 to 50 cm long and a small chamber 10 to 15 cm in diameter, more or less filled with litter. It consists of rice straw, hay, leaves green or dead, mainly of guava trees, or of papers, rags or various finely nibbled scraps. The litter condition is a good indicator of the age of the burrow and its degree of use. It is not uncommon to discover, among all kinds of residue, skulls or fragments of rat skeletons or tufts of their fur; in the case of treatment by rat poison, there are whole corpses there. In the absence of hosts or newly fed fleas, the best index of occupancy of the nest is provided by the existence of a particular biocenotic fauna, where small mesostigmata mites (Macrochelidae) are dominant. In the inhabited litter, these little mites swarm; in abandoned litter, however, they are absent or rare, whereas spring-tails, pseudo-scorpions, woodlice, ants, and spiders are numerous. In this bio-tope, there is still a lack of carnivorous larvae of Coleoptera, which among other fauna are the main predators of flea larvae.
>
> (Klein 1966:7)

Although the original group of rats in the burrow may abandon the site, particu-larly after pups leave the nest, the structures are not permanently abandoned. Rats passing through the area may use the nests and caches in the burrows 'cassava stores, passageways or places of consumption' (Klein 1966: 7). On sites particularly favourable to the life of the rat, due to the nearness and 'abundance of food sources, terrain relief, irrigation continuous and a cover of guavas', large sets of burrows will be maintained year after year by different rat groups (ibid.). The burrow systems are useful to other species as well. Klein also observed that abandoned nests are often used by highly plague-resistant greater hedgehog tenrecs (*Setifer sefosus*), an endemic species in Madagascar considered by the Malagasy to be delectable game.

The question of whether potentially infectious fleas occupy rat burrows in the absence of rats can be partly answered by Klein's findings, although he discovered only dead fleas and was not testing for *Y. pestis* in burrows. He notes fleas are only found in galleries that rats abandoned (Klein 1966: 8). Regarding the relationship between the burrow system, flea reproduction, and plague transmission, Klein suggests that 'the degree of occupation and the age of the burrows, the state of the nesting litter and the presence of predators, which explain the large variations observed' (ibid.: 20). As in the case of prairie dog burrows, co-travelled by ground squirrels and fleas, fleas in abandoned galleries present the opportunity for plague transmission to other individuals.

Burrow systems shed light on how *Y. pestis* has probably travelled in networks at different spatial strata, on the surface in vehicles of various sorts, and under-ground in multispecies bodies. Recent scientific studies of burrow systems have evolved out of earlier theories about the transmissibility and recrudescence of the plague through the soil (Lynteris 2017b).

As mentioned previously, scientists' interest in rodent structures emerged as early as the twentieth century, not yet as a distinct object of scientific analysis but as pertinent ethnographic detail. In his study of plague outbreaks on the Russian-Chinese frontier at the turn of the twentieth century, Lynteris (2016) describes the ways in which scientists theorised plague transmission mechanisms with fragments of ethnographic information about marmot-human relations, marmots being plague's host species in the region and an important protein source for indigenous people. He argues that scientists formulated a theory about plague's emergence in the region based on presumed differences in expertise about marmot hunting between migrant and indigenous people. Scientists had accepted ethnographic lore that indigenous Buryat and Mongol hunters could identify healthy versus pestiferous marmots, whereas migrants could not. Indigenous hunters were therefore thought to have developed precautionary hunting techniques to avoid infection.

What Lynteris calls the 'native knowledge hypothesis' was built upon a foundational piece of ethnographic writing by Russian explorer, Gustave Ferdinand Richard Radde, who undertook an expedition of Siberia in 1857. Radde wrote down cultural practices of the people he encountered. In one passage, he describes how 'pagan hunters' would hit the ground above burrows with pick-axes to scare the animals out of their holes, or would seal and smoke up holes to suffocate the animals in their nests (Lynteris 2016: 45). This piece and other ethnographic claims about cultural knowledge and practice were largely unsubstantiated and even contradictory, Lynteris argues. Yet they reveal an adjustment of the scientific gaze, a view of disease transmission as species jump. Moreover, these claims reflect an emergent understanding of soils as construction material for burrowing animals in which a plague-harbouring architecture takes shape, rather than as solely a medium of bacterial propogation.

Plague arrives in Madagascar

Plague arrived suddenly in Madagascar by ship in 1898. It has been assumed, and is often retold in scholarly publications, that an infected ship sailed into the port of Tamatave directly from India. But the actual series of events was more roundabout and unusual.

The source of the epidemic had been a Madagascar-based passenger steamship, *La Gironde*, travelling from the island to Mozambique in mid-November 1898. The steamship made contact on the open sea with a ship of the British East India Company (presumably heading south from India). According to a report sent to Paris by the Governor General of Madagascar, Maréchal Galliéni, this ship was infected with plague, and somehow while at sea the disease jumped (via rats?) from the British ship to *La Gironde* (Galliéni 1898).

Galliéni received a cablegram on November 17 informing him that *La Gironde* was not permitted to discharge in Mozambique because a doctor, the head of the sanitary service at the port, 'seemed to have not the slightest doubt' that a corpse and a patient on board were infected with the plague. The next day, three more cases emerged. *La Gironde* turned around and headed back to Madagascar with five sick passengers on board. Galliéni ordered the captain to avoid all contact with land and to remain in quarantine for nine days in the bay of Diego Suarez. But then his report to Paris becomes somewhat ambiguous. He writes that the 'gravity of the news' they had received from Mozambique was greatly lightened by news sent from Diego Suarez.

A cablegram sent to Tamatave by the doctor, the head of sanitary services at the port of Diego Suarez, had reported the following:

> Urgent. 'Ville du Havre' just arrived in Diego with a clean bill of health and was granted free pratique. Here is all the information given by the captain: 'Gironde anchored in Diego on the morning of the 20th. One hour after the Ville du Havre left, the boarding of Gironde not yet finished, but captain learns there was a deceased on board [whose death] would have been attributed to beriberi'.
>
> (Galliéni 1898)

Galliéni appears to believe that the earlier cablegram from Mozambique had been a 'false alarm'. The ship was allowed to proceed southward along the east coastline to Tamatave. A plague outbreak erupted on the main commercial avenue on November 22, 1898 (see also: Lhuerre 1937; Keorner 1994: 454).

Mifflin Wister Gibbs, a United States Consul to Madagascar at that time, recounts in his autobiography his impressions of Tamatave on the day he arrived in Madagascar, several months before the outbreak (Gibbs 1995 [1902]). When he disembarked at the port, he was struck by its insalubrious state. At the time, Tamatave was a hub of foreign diplomacy and trade in the recently annexed French colony.

In Gibbs' eyes, the alarm of the plague outbreak in November prompted favourable changes for the town. Galliéni implemented a raft of sanitation and beautification measures, emulating efforts elsewhere in the imperial network (Brygoo 1966). At the time, the prevailing scientific knowledge of plague was that it could fester in waste, grains, and other material objects, and could be harboured in soils. Following the protocol for outbreaks practiced elsewhere at the time, Galliéni imposed sanitary cordons around Tamatave to limit traffic to and from the outbreak epicentre. People and goods were quarantined. Buildings and effects were burned and/or sprayed with chemical disinfectants.

Authorities in Tamatave were invested in creating a firm barrier between people's feet and the contaminated soil. Paving roads, sidewalks, and creeks; directing rain water into gutters, drainage systems, and out to sea; and managing the seepage of waste into the ground water were part of the plan, as Mr Ernest Pontzen, civil engineer, explains in a committee report:

> The suppression of the use of wells, taking water from the water table that extends under the town, is not immediately possible; it is enough to do away with the use of permeable pits into which people throw dirty water and fecal

material. We will redress the contamination of underground water. There is an interest in moving forward with the implementation of a clean water supply in Tamatave. Following that, we will recommend the removal of wells in houses.

(Pontzen 1899)

In addition, roads were widened (in part because rats avoid exposure on large roads), plans for a clean water supply were drawn up, floors and walls were cemented, and a method of drying, pulverising, and storing fecal matter in more sanitary pans (*tinettes*) was introduced.

Major transportation projects were also being launched at the time. The state recruited Malagasy labourers to build a vehicular road between Tamatave and the capital, as well as a railway line (Frémagacci 2006). Both required penetrating the thick, mountainous rainforest. Both enabled the wide dispersion of plague-carrying rats along these corridors. Furthermore, the road and railway cut opened up the rainforest to Malagasy cultivators, attracting rats into newly established villages.

Although this hygienic regime may have improved the quality of life for many, it was not foolproof against plague. The last cases of the first outbreak ended in early February 1989. A second outbreak flared up in July 1899. 'Foul surroundings are recognised as hotbeds for the propagation of the germs of this pest', Gibbs writes, yet 'cleanliness and rigid sanitary measures . . . are not positive barriers to its approach and dire effect' (Gibbs 1995 [1902]: 242).

Plague had implanted a chronic sense of dreadful possibility. The first plague outbreak resulted in 288 cases and 197 deaths, including 101 Malagasy, 39 Creoles and Metis, 56 Indians, and 1 European. The tally indicated an uneven flow of bacteria to distinct ethnic groups, chalked up by colonial scientists to the degree of cleanliness of various quarters of town. The 1899 outbreak resulted in a more favourable outcome overall: fifty-two cases and forty-two deaths, with the vast proportion of deaths still being Malagasy, and, again, one European (Anonymous 1901; Koerner 1994). By this point, rats had become targets for eradication:

Rats, considered the main promoter of the disease, Tamatave inhabitants are still strongly urged to destroy the animals. Rats caught in traps should be killed by boiling water and sent from between 7–9 am, or 3–5 pm, to the agent responsible for destroying them by fire, at the place between the slaughterhouse and the railway line, by the sea, behind the village of Ampassimazava. A sum of .25 franc will be given for each rat reported. It is recommended to avoid touching the rats.

(Anonymous 1899)

Plague incrementally made its way westward to the central highland capital of Antananarivo by 1921, a region known as Imerina and inhabited by the Merina ethnic population. An outbreak killed forty-eight family members who attended a wedding party. The pathogen gradually fanned outward from there (Esoavelomandroso 1981: 168).

Georges Girard, head of the Pasteur Institute in Antananarivo from 1922 to 1950, believed that the capital's relative isolation from the coasts had spared it from plague outbreak until the completion of the railway in 1913 (Girard 1951; Coulanges 1982). The disease crept gradually westward to higher elevations, from the port of Tamatave, 'as evidenced by murine epizootic area discovered at the time in Périnet (Andasibe) near Moramanga' (Chanteau et al. 2006: 42).

Over time, the plague established various strains in different phylogenetic groups of rats (Tollenaere et al. 2010; Vogler et al. 2017). Plague's persistence on the island is most likely explained by local transmission cycles, rather than the translocation of one plague-carrying rat subpopulation to new area, which has occasionally occurred through human modes of transport (Vogler et al. 2017). Local transmission cycles are buttressed by burrow systems, whose ranges appear to be limited by landscape barriers.

Malagasy historian Farinirina Esoavelomandroso (1981: 174) writes that in the capital, the 1921 outbreak of pneumonic plague, when the disease was transmitted in an airborne manner, compelled the state to implement draconian measures, starting with a sanitary cordon around the city. Authorities burned dwellings, applied chemical disinfectants and raticide, and rat-proofed new constructions. In 1925, the state required all new buildings to have foundations and basements made of hard materials, such as concrete and cement, to 'prevent the natural shelters of rats'. The new housing policy called for the allotment of community-owned terrain to those whose homes had been incinerated. Expelled occupants would get a land parcel to build a home that had to comply with the new building code (ibid.: 174–175).

Among other deeply unpopular hygienic measures were rules governing the burial of plague victims. The state prohibited the Malagasy practice of *famadihana*, a ritual signifying 'secondary burial' and the means by which the realm of the living is clearly separated from the realm of ancestors (Bloch 1993 [1971]; see also: McGeorge 1974). Ethnic populations around the island practice *famadihana*, with variations in content and symbolism. Within Merina communities of the highlands, the ritual involves opening the family tomb, exhuming the bodies that had sufficiently decomposed, and rewrapping bones in a new burial shroud. People clack the bones overhead while dancing in celebration of the person's life before placing the deceased back on the 'bed' of the tomb (Raison-Jourde 1983; Razafindralambo 2005).

Poleykett (2018) explains that for plague victims, authorities believed that exhuming the remains of plague victims (one to several years after death) risked infecting people with still active bacteria. To ensure that *famadihana* would not be performed for plague victims who were still infectious, Girard recommended the delay of the ritual for three years (Esoavelomandroso 1981: 178). His reasoning was based on a series of laboratory experiments on infected fleas, after which he 'concluded that if the dead were disinterred prematurely, infection could take place as plague infected fleas could live, breed, and feed in the tombs for several months' (Poleykett 2018: 6).

The colonial state had by 1933 updated legislation to reflect current Pasteurian science regarding the infectivity of human remains. The pestiferous dead were to be buried in separate cemeteries. The state added 'a dispensation', however, making it 'possible for natives wishing to carry out a "provisional burial". This could be accomplished if another tomb was installed to the side of the family tomb, as long as this tomb was constructed of "solid and hermetic masonry" and was impervious to rats' (Poleykett 2018: 8–9; Archives Nationales de Madagascar n.d.).

Not until 1935 did scientists in Antananarivo find an effective vaccine against the plague, called the E.V. vaccine (from a family name, Evesque, but known familiarly by Malagasy as 'Enfant Vazaha', or 'white people's child') (Coulanges 1982: 175). The vaccine offered protection against the bubonic plague but only temporarily. As a later director of the Pasteur Institute of Madagascar, Edouard R. Brygoo, declared, it was a 'palliative', but did not 'attack the reservoir' of the germ (ibid.; 178).

When Brygoo took over as director of the Pasteur Institute of Madagascar in 1964 (after having served as deputy director for a decade), he stopped some of the more contentious policies advised by his predecessors, particularly the enforced vaccination of the general population. He instead recommended outbreak surveillance, the use of DDT to eradicate fleas from homes, and treatment with streptomycin, as Poleykett recounts. Brygoo aimed to 'attenuate the symbolic power of the plague' for Malagasy people, to render the disease common (Poleykett 2018: 10). Brygoo envisioned that by softening its approach to plague control, the state might begin to change Malagasy people's resistance to biomedical authority. Resistance to the treatment of corpses and to burial policies had induced many Malagasy subjects to hide their plague dead and to distrust scientific medical treatments.

During Brygoo's term with the Pasteur Institute, which ended in 1972, plague had virtually been tamped out in Antananarivo. The disease reemerged there in 1979, but outbreaks continued to mostly crop up in the rural periphery (Andrianaivoarimanana et al. 2013: 2). The large outbreak of pneumonic and bubonic plague in 2017 was brought in from outside the city.

The disease dynamics of urban plague had indeed changed due to architectural changes and sanitary measures, but not because rats had been foiled. Rodent surveillance carried out in the 1990s revealed that over time, the black rat (also known as 'roof rat' or 'ship rat'), which prefers thatched roofs and rafters, had been overtaken in the city by the larger, partly aquatic brown rat (*Rattus norvegicus*), also known as the 'street rat' or 'sewer rat' (Duplantier et al. 2005). The shift in building materials from wood and mud to concrete and stone prevented tunnelling by black rats, while the construction of a modern sewage system provided an agreeable space for brown rats (Duplantier et al. 2005: 441). The colonisation of the city by brown rats, which are highly plague-resistant, diminished the frequency of rat epizootics and therefore human plague outbreaks.

Burials and burrows

While Brygoo ended the coercive vaccination campaign, he apparently never advised officials of Independent Madagascar to change policies concerning the burial of plague victims. Pasteur Institute scientists today cannot find reference to the exact legal code, but they disseminate guidelines from the Ministry of Health about how to handle plague deaths: disinfect and bag the bodies; place bodies in separate, designated grave sites for a period of seven years (rather than the three years under Girard) in order to ensure the delay of *famadihana*; and dig pits twelve metres deep in order to reach hard ground.

These guidelines recall the historical theories about infectious corpses and soils (Lynteris and Evans 2018). Yet today, the risk of rat burrows penetrating plague pits justifies the policy. To date, however, no one has conducted a study in Madagascar to determine how long *Y. pestis* survives in corpses (Andrianaivoarimananana et al. 2013).

Ethnographic findings in Moramanga District, where I am investigating the cultural impacts of a 2015 plague outbreak, illustrate how ideas of rat infrastructure have 'burrowed' into Malagasy funerary practices and eschatology (Ramasindrazana et al. 2017). The Moramanga District lies approximately 72 miles east of the capital. Most residents identify ethnically as Bezanozano and Betsimisaraka and practice subsistence agriculture. They plant paddy rice on lowlands and burn forest and vegetation to plant hill rice. The frequency of their encounters with rats depends on the phase of the agricultural cycle. Village homes are made predominantly of red earth and dung with thatched roofs (*rojopeta*). Numerous rat tunnels perforate the bases of *rojopeta* (see Figure 6.1), which people repeatedly plug.

Rats tend to be more abundant in rice fields and the sisal hedges that border them during the ripening of the rice crop, but flea populations boom later in the season. Humans are at greater risk of plague infection when the flea population is abundant, and rats are scarce, a population shift that may be indicative of,an epizootic kill-off (Rahelinirina et al. 2010: 80). Up until very recently, the plague season spanned September to November. However, climate change has altered the reproductive cycles of both rats and fleas and therefore altered the plague's seasonality (Andrianaivoarimanana et al. 2013: 2). For the past few years, outbreaks in Moramanga District have occurred in August.

Familial tombs in this region vary in structure. For some families, the deceased are inserted into caves in the forest, and bodies are sex-separated. It is also common to find large communal graves in which several bodies, wrapped in burial shrouds (*lamba*) are laid side-by-side, and tiers are added as needed over time. The base of the pit is lined with wooden planks, and another layer of planks are placed over the bodies. In the town of Moramanga, one sees cemeteries containing expensive cement tombs shaped like small houses, the type more common around the capital.

In the hamlets struck by plague in 2015, people buried their dead (the ones who did not die in the hospital) in familial tombs or individual graves, depending on the status of the deceased. Mrs. Matana describes the burial of her 22-year-old son, who died in the August 2015 outbreak:

> The funeral went as follows. We bought a white cloth in Moramanga, then had a wake at night, then buried him the next day. There was only us there, the family, at the burial. . . . A grave of about 2.5 meters deep was dug, then

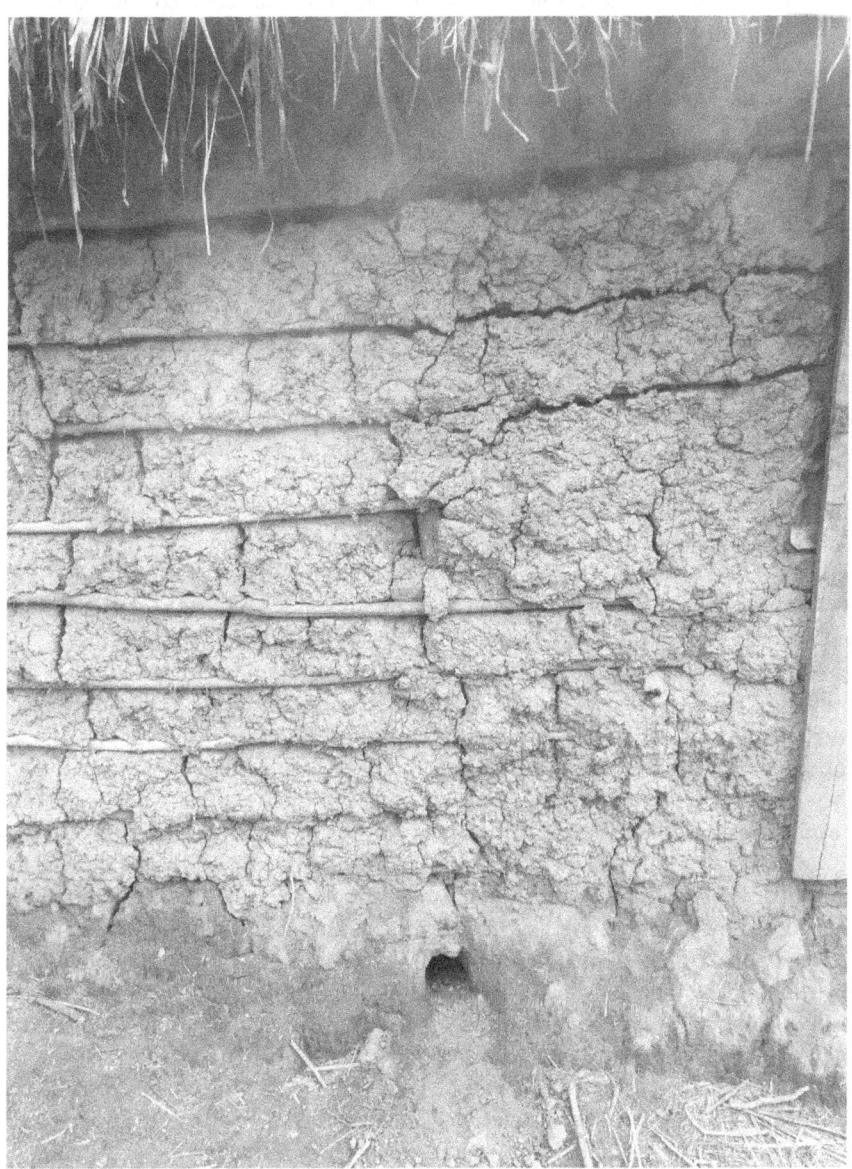

Figure 6.1 Rat tunnel at base of mud-and-dung home in Moramanga District
Photograph by Genese Marie Sodikoff, 2017

covered on the bottom with wooden planks. The body was already wrapped in white cloth and then placed in the grave with the head facing the north. Afterwards, a plank was laid on top and the grave was covered with earth.

Actually, we are all immigrants in the region, since we all come from Kakato. We plan on transporting the body to our ancestral land as soon as we can. There was no song, no shots of rum during the wake. Only us two, crying. At 7:00 am, we buried the body, asking for help, but no one wanted to help us because everyone was afraid of the plague. A little time later, a declaration [about the plague] was made in the quarter of Antsahatsihanarina, and this paper is still posted.

(Fieldnotes, 7/2016)

Family members who buried victims of the 2015 outbreak in individual graves did so as a temporary measure. They intend to save up funds to repatriate the remains to their ancestral land, as Mrs. Matana explained previously, or to afford to buy a zebu (*Bos taurus indicus*), which must be sacrificed only upon opening the tomb to deposit a corpse. If buried bodies have been subjected to the seven-year waiting period (that is, if the victims died in hospital rather than the village), the family must wait to sacrifice a zebu until the transfer of remains to the tomb takes place. To do so prematurely is called 'dancing before the umbilical cord is cut' (*mandihy tsy afa-tavony*), alluding to the liminal state of adults exiled in plague pits who have had their first burial but not the momentous second one. They are dead but yet not ancestors in the true sense.

A middle-aged couple, Jean-Paul and Baotine, assumed responsibility for bringing their sick relatives to the local health clinic or more distant hospital in Moramanga town, as well as buying a sacrificial zebu and other funeral provisions for one their relatives, who died of plague in the village. The couple related that they were not permitted to bring home the bodies of four relatives who died in the hospital. Instead, the hospital staff slid the corpses into plastic sacks and drove a few miles away to deposit the bodies in a potter's field. The couple was allowed to accompany the staffers, and Jean-Paul was instructed to help dig the pit, but they were not allowed to perform any funerary rites or leave any offerings.

The bodies (three men and one woman), were lain in a pit approximately 1.5 metres deep, without any wooden planks to protect the bodies from the earth below, or rain above, explained Jean-Paul and Baotine returned a short time later with a blue plastic tarp to cover the grave. Jean-Paul remembers the hospital orderlies being in a great hurry to leave the site, and the whole process was rushed.

Dr Minoarisoa Rajerison, head of plague unit at the Pasteur Institute, relayed to me that the official guidelines for plague graves. They should be dug to a depth of

around twelve meters, but this is not always respected and is often not so easy. In certain areas, even at two meters deep you reach the water table, and you can't dig any deeper. What is strongly demanded is to dig a sort of drawer into [the side] of the pit, where one slides in the corpse.

(Personal communication, January 29, 2018)

Since digging approximately 36 feet into hard earth with shovels and spades is impractical and exhausting, the guidelines are routinely ignored. Dr Minoarisoa Rajerison and Dr Beza Ramansindraza, mammalogist at the Pasteur Institute, explained during an interview in August 2017 that excessive depth of the pit and additional 'drawer' are meant to prevent the possibility (admittedly unlikely) of rats burrowing toward the infectious corpses and absorbing plague bacteria.

Pasteur Institute scientists do not enforce rules, but they take an epidemiological interest in knowing about compliance. Their belief in, or at least refusal to dismiss, the potential of rat burrows as conduits toward infectious corpses and repositories of active plague reflects the extent to the plague in Madagascar remains in many ways mysterious.

Conclusion

Scholars have argued that urban infrastructure has been formative of modern subjectivity by connecting disparate social groups, imposing state biopower, shaping the sensorium of city life, liberating human energies, and so on. But what kind of subjectivities do pathogenic infrastructures engender?

I have suggested that many material infrastructures are intrinsically multispecies, and their multispecies quality becomes apparent during the anxious times of outbreak. However, zoonotic disease infrastructures are more than human, and their multispecies dimensions matter to the public health.

By 1898, once the decisive role of rats and fleas in plague transmission became widely accepted, scientists and officials themselves began to perceive human-made infrastructure through a multispecies lens, and began directing attention to rodent-built crawlways that might play a role in plague transmission. Urban plague control, once focused on the sanitisation of the ground underfoot, shifted to an emphasis on rat-and-flea control. States recruited rat-disposal agents in plague-struck towns. They implemented rat-proofing ordinances for buildings, waste disposal sites, and food storage facilities. They sought to prevent the transport of infected rats overland and overseas through sanitary cordons, quarantines, and the fumigation of ships.

In urban centres of Madagascar, these measures, alongside vaccination and education campaigns, suppressed plague outbreaks for decades, even while Malagasy tried to subvert the system to protect the wellbeing of their dead. In Antananarivo, the installation of modern sewer lines and changes in building and tomb construction reconfigured the plague's ecology. The city became less inviting to black rats and more conducive to colonisation by plague-resistant brown rats, thereby lessening the frequency of zoonotic encounters.

In the rural central highlands, however, black rat populations established extensive burrow systems at the edges of agricultural fields and amidst mud-walled houses. In Moramanga District, where outbreaks resurge with increasing regularity, this animal-built infrastructure of the plague not only harbours bacteria in rat and flea bodies but also indirectly damages residents' relationship to deceased ancestors. Unresolved since the early colonial era, questions about the infectiousness of corpses compel medical scientists and officials today to maintain repressive burial policies. The architecture of rural homes and graves is perceived as vulnerable to plague due to the subterranean structures of rats. Medical scientists surmise that if plague can survive underground in decomposing flesh and soil microbes, rats can potentially absorb bacteria by tunnelling towards the corpse. The multispecies quality of burrow systems, which link rodent subpopulations and harbour infectious fleas, appears indeed to support the plague's underground survival. As a corollary, burrow systems, by forging imagined routes between rats and buried kin, also link marginalised rural communities to the state in undesirable ways. Due to their hypothetical role as disease conduits, rat burrows justify the state's precautionary measures for plague deaths, thereby sustaining rural people's resistance to an authority that meddles with their obligations to ancestors.

Note

1 Kreppel et al. (2016) suggest that *S. fonquerniei* is better adapted to cooler climate compared to *X. cheopis*, which has enabled it 'sustain the plague cycle throughout the cold season where temperatures fall below 18°C inside rat burrows until the population of *X. cheopis* is thriving again in the warm summer months'.

References

Archival Sources Archives Nationales de Madagascar Campagne Anti Pesteuse, H293 (n.d.).
Galliéni, Maréchal 'Rapport Politique, Arrêtes et Circulaires', FR ANOM FP/44PA/carton 5, dossier 29, No. 3992 A, p. 9 (November 29,1898).
Pontzen, Ernest 'Comité des Travaux Publics des Colonies, Séance du 4 mai 1899, Rapport de la Commission', FR ANOM FM 1 TP, carton 343, dossier 3 (April 27, 1899).

Published sources

Anand, Nikhil *Hydraulic City: Water and the Infrastructures of Citizenship in Mumbai* (Durham, NC: Duke University Press, 2017).
Andrianaivoarimanana, Voahangy, Sandra Telfer, Minoarisoa Rajerison, Michel A. Ranjalahy, Fehivola Andriamiarimanana, Corinne Rahaingosoamamitiana, Lila Rahalison, and Ronan Jambou 'Immune responses to plague infection in wild *Rattus rattus*', *PLOS Neglected Tropical Diseases* (June 18, 2012). https://doi.org/10.1371/journal.pone.0038630
Andrianaivoarimanana, Voahangy, Katharina Kreppel, Nohal Elissa, Jean-Marc Duplantier, Elisabeth Carniel, Minoarisoa Rajerison, and Ronan Jambou 'Understanding the persistence of plague foci in Madagascar', *PLOS Neglected Tropical Diseases* (November 7, 2013). https://doi.org/10.1371/journal.pntd.0002382
Anonymous 'The relative importance of various agencies in the propagation of the Plague', *Public Health Reports (1896–1970)* 15 (7) (February 16, 1900), 319–322.
Anonymous 'France. Measures taken at Tamatave and at Antsirane (Madagascar), against plague that occurred in these two localities during the year 1899', *Public Health Reports (1896–1970)* 16 (6) (February 8, 1901), 267–268.

Anonymous 'Exterminating rats to stamp out the black death: How science is waging a war to keep the bubonic plague from making its period girdle of the earth', *New York Times* (November 20, 1910). SM7.

Anonymous 'Ship rats and plague', *Public Heath Reports (1896–1970)* 29 (16) (April 17, 1914), 927–928.

Anonymous Report from Mayor's Office 'La peste à Madagascar (1899): Situation sanitaire de Tamatave', *Journal official de Madagascar et Dépendences*. Supplément Comercial (Tamatave et Côte Est (September 20, 1899)). Actualité Culturelle Malgache. http://cultmada.blogspot.com/

Blanchy, Sixte 'Contribution de l'histoire à la comprehension de l'épidémiologie de la peste à Madagascar', *Histore des Sciences Médicales* 29 (4) (1995), 355–364.

Bloch, Maurice *Placing the Dead: Tombs, Ancestral Villages, and Kinship Organization in Madagascar* (Long Grove, IL: Waveland Press Inc., 1993 [1971]).

Brouat, Carine, Soanandrasana Rahelinirina, Anne Loiseau, Lila Rahalison, Minoariso Rajerison, Dominque Laffly, Pascal Handschumacher, and Jean-Marc Duplantier 'Plague circulation and population genetics of the reservoir *Rattus rattus*: The influence of topographic relief on the distribution of the disease within the Madagascan focus', *PLoS Neglected Tropical Diseases* 7 (6) (2013), e2266. DOI:10.1371/journal.pntd.0002266

Brown, Hannah, and Ann H. Kelly 'Material proximities and hotspots: Toward an anthropology of viral hemorrhagic fevers', *Medical Anthropology Quarterly* 28 (2) (2014), 280–303.

Brygoo, E. R. 'Epidemiologie de la peste a Madagascar', *Archives de l'Institut Pasteur de Madagascar* 35 (1966), 1–219.

Buell, Paul D. 'Qubilai and the rats', *Sudhoffs Archiv: Zeitschrift für Wissensch* 96 (2) (2012), 127–144.

Chanteau, Suzanne C., Pascal Boiser, Elisabeth Carniel, Jean Bernard Duchemin, Jean Marc Duplantier, Steve M. Goodman, Pascal Hanschumacher, Isabelle Jeanne, Stephane Laventure, Philippe Mauclère, René Miglianai, Dieudonné Rabeson, Lila Rahalison, Noelson Rasolofonirina, Lala Rasifasoamanana, Bruno Rasoamanana, Maherisoa Ratsitorahina, Jocelyn Ratovonjato, Marie Laure Rosso, Jean Roux, and Adama Tall *Atlas de la peste à Madagascar* (Paris: Institut de Recherche pour le Développement, Institut Pasteur, Agence Universitaire de la Francophonie, 2006).

Chu, Julie Y. 'When infrastructures attack: The workings of disrepair in China', *American Ethnologist* 41 (2) (2014), 351–367.

Coulanges, P. 'Cinquantenaire du vaccin antipesteux EV. (Girard et Robica)', *Archives Institut Pasteur Madagascar* 50 (1) (1982), 169–184.

Dourish, Paul, and Genevieve Bell 'The Infrastructure of experience and the experience of infrastructure: Meaning and structure in everyday encounters with space', *Environment and Planning B: Urban Analytics and City Science* 34 (2007), 414–430.

Duchemin, Jean-Bernard *Biogéographie des puces de Madagascar*. Doctoral Thesis. Université de Paris XII – Val de Marne, Faculté de Médecine de Créteil Ecole doctorale: Sciences de la Vie et de la Santé Interaction Hôtes-Parasites, 2003.

Duplantier, Jean-Marc, Jean-Bernard Duchemin, Suzanne Chanteau, and Elisabeth Carniel 'From the recent lessons of the Malagasy foci towards a global understanding of the factors involved in plague reemergence', *Veterinary Research* 36 (2005), 437–453. DOI: 10.1051/vetres:2005007

Echenberg, Myron 'Pestis redux: The initial years of the third bubonic plague pandemic, 1894–1901', *Journal of World History* 13 (2) (2002), 429–449.

Echenberg, Myron *Plague Ports: The Global Urban Impact of Bubonic Plague 1894–1901* (New York: New York University Press, 2007).

Elyachar, Julia 'Phatic labor, infrastructure, and the question of empowerment in Cairo', *American Ethnologist* 37 (3) (2010), 452–464.

Engelmann, Lukas 'Fumigating the hygienic model city: Bubonic plague and the Sulfurozador in early-twentieth-century Buenos Aires', *Medical History* 62 (3) (2018), 360–382.

Esoavelomandroso, Faranirina 'Résistance à la médecine en situation coloniale: La peste à Madagascar', *Annales. Histoire, Sciences Sociales* 36e Année (2) (March–April 1981), 168–190.

Evans, Nicholas H. A. 'Blaming the Rat? Accounting for plague in colonial Indian medicine', *Medicine, Anthropology, Theory* 5 (3) (2018), 15–42.

Fleischer, Jodi, Rick Yarborough, Jeff Piper, and Steve Jones 'Rat population increase can have real impact on city infrastructure', *NBC4 News4 I Team* (August 11, 2017). www. nbcwashington.com/investigations/Rat-Increase-Can-Have-Real-Impact-on-City-Infra structure-439698493.html

Frémagacci, Jean 'Les chemins de fer de Madagascar (1901–1936): Une modernisation manquée', *Afrique et Histoire* 2 (6) (2006), 161–191.

Friggens, Megan M., Robert R. Parmenter, Michael Boyden, Paulette L. Ford, Kenneth Gage, and Paul Keim 'Flea abundance, diversity, and plague in Gunnison's prairie dogs (*Cynomys Gunnisoni*) and their burrows in montane grasslands in northern New Mexico', *Journal of Wildlife Diseases* 46 (2) (2010), 356–367.

Gibbs, Mifflin Wistar *Shadow and Light: An Autobiography with Reminiscences of the Last and Present Century*. Introduction by Booker T. Washington. (Lincoln, NB: University of Nebraska Press, 1995 [1902]).

Girard, G. 'La peste: Contribution apportée par Madagascar à l'état actuel de nos connaissances', *Revue Coloniale de Médecine et de Chirogie* 25 (1951), 138–144.

Girard, G., and F. Estrade 'Nouvelle observation de peste dans un élevage de lapins et de cobayes consécutive à une épizootic murine', *Bulletin de la Société de Pathologie Exotique* 27 (1934), 962–963.

Klein, Jean-Marie 'Données écologiques et biologiques sur *Synopsyllus fonquerniei* Wagner et Roubaud, 1932 (*Siphonaptera*), puce du rat péridomestique, dans la région de Tananarive', *Cahiers ORSTOM, Série Entomologie Médicale et Parasitologie* 4 (1966), 3–29.

Koerner, F. 'La protection sanitaire des populations à Madagascar (1862–1914)', *Revue Historique* T. 291, Fasc. 2 (590) (1994), 439–458.

Kosoy, Michael, and Karen Bakker 'Technologies of government: Constituting subjectivities, spaces, and infrastructures in colonial and contemporary Jakarta', *International Journal of Urban and Regional Research* 32 (2) (2008), 375–391.

Kreppel, Katharina S., Cyril Caminade, Sandra Telfer, Minoarison Rajerison, Lila Rahalison, Andy Morse, and Matthew Baylis 'A non-stationary relationship between global climate phenomena and human plague incidence in Madagascar', *PLOS Neglected Tropical Diseases* 8 (10) (2014), e3155. DOI:10.1371/journal.pntd.0003155

Kreppel, Katharina S., Sandra Telfer, Minorisoa Rajerison, Andy Morse, and Matthew Baylis 'Effect of temperature and relative humidity on the development times and survival of *Synopsyllus fonquerniei* and *Xenopsylla cheopis*, the flea vectors of plague in Madagascar', *Parasites and Vectors* 9 (82) (2016). https://doi.org/10.1186/s13071-016-1366-z

Larkin, Brian *Signal and Noise: Infrastructure, and Urban Culture in Nigeria* (Durham, NC: Duke University Press, 2008)

Larkin, Brian 'The politics and poetics of infrastructure', *Annual Review of Anthropology* 42 (2013), 327–343. https://doi.org/10.1146/annurev-anthro-092412-155522

Lefebvre, Henri *The Production of Space*, translated by Donald Nicholson-Smith (Oxford: Wiley-Blackwell, 1991 (1974]).

Lhuerre, R. *Le paludisme et la peste à Madagascar (influence des climats, des races, des mœurs)*. Thèse de doctorat en médecine, Lyon (1937).

Little, Lester 'Review article: Plague historians in lab coats', *Past and Present* 213 (2011), 267–290.

Lynteris, Christos 'Skilled natives, inept coolies: Marmot hunting and the great Manchurian pneumonic plague (1910–1911)', *History and Anthropology* 24 (3) (2013), 303–321.

Lynteris, Christos *Ethnographic Plague: Configuring Disease on the Chinese-Russian Frontier* (London: Palgrave Macmillan, 2016).

Lynteris, Christos 'Zoonotic diagrams: Mastering and unsettling human-animal relations', *Journal of the Royal Anthropological Institute* (N.S.) 23 (2017a), 463–485.

Lynteris, Christos 'A "suitable soil": Plague's urban breeding grounds at the dawn of the third pandemic', *Medical History* 61 (3) (2017b), 343–357.

Lynteris, Christos, and Nicholas H. A. Evans 'Introduction: The challenge of the epidemic corpse', In Christos Lynteris, and Nicholas H. A. Evans (eds.), *Histories of Post-Mortem Contagion: Infectious Corpses and Contested Burials*, pp. 1–26 (London: Palgrave Macmillan, 2018).

McCormick, Michael 'Rats, communications, and plague: Toward an ecological history', *The Journal of Interdisciplinary History* 34 (1) (2003), 1–25.

McGeorge, Susan 'Imerina Famadihana as a secondary burial', *Achipel* 7 (1974), 21–39.

Miarinjara, Adélaïde, Jean Vergain, Jean Marcel Kavaruganda, Minoarisoa Rajerison, and Sébastien Boyer 'Plague risk in vulnerable community: Assessment of Xenopsylla cheopis susceptibility to insecticides in Malagasy prisons', *Infectious Diseases of Poverty* 6 (141) (2017), 1–7.

Morita, Atsuro 'Multispecies infrastructure: Infrastructural inversion and involutionary entanglements in the Chao Phraya Delta, Thailand', *Ethnos* 82 (4) (2017), 738–757.

Poleykett, Branwyn 'Ethnohistory and the dead: Cultures of colonial epidemiology', *Medical Anthropology* (2018). DOI:10.1080/01459740.2018.1453507

Rahelinirina, Soanandrasana, Jean Marc Duplantier, Jocelyn Ratovonjato, Olga Ramilijaona, Mamy Ratsimba, and Lila Rahalison 'Study on the movement of *Rattus rattus* and evaluation of the plague dispersion in Madagascar', *Vector-Borne and Zoonotic Diseases* 10 (1) (2010), 77–84.

Raison-Jourde, Françoise *Les souverains de Madagascar* (Paris: Karthala Editions, 1983).

Ramasindrazana, Beza, Voahangy Andrianaivoarimanana, Jean Marius Rakotondramanga, Dawn N. Birdsell, Mahcrisoa Ratsitorahina, and Minoarisoa Rajerison 'Pneumonic plague transmission, Moramanga, Madagascar, 2015', *Emerging Infectious Diseases* 23 (3) (2017), 521–524.

Razafindralambo, L.N. 'Inégalités, exclusion, représentations sur les Hautes Terres centrales de Madagascar', *Cahiers d'Etudes Africaines* 45 (179/180) (2005), 879–903.

Rucker, W.C. 'Plague: The relation between traffic and the spread of plague', *Public Health Reports (1896–1970)* 28 (4) (January 24, 1913), 163–166.

Schmid, B. B., M. Jesse, L. I. Wilschut, H. Viljugrein, J. A. P. Heesterbeek 'Local persistence and extinction of plague in a metapopulation of great gerbil burrows, Kazakhstan', *Epidemics* 4 (4) (2012), 211–218.

Simond, Marc, Margaret L. Godley, and Pierre D. E. Mouriquand 'Paul-Louis Simond and his discovery of plague transmission by rat fleas: A centenary', *Journal of the Royal Society of Medicine* 91 (2) (1998), 101–104.

Simond, Paul-Louis 'La propagation de la peste' *Annales de l'Institut Pasteur* 12 (1898), 625–687.

Simone, AbdouMaliq 'People as infrastructure: Intersecting fragments in Johannesburg', *Public Culture* 16 (3) (2004), 407–429.

Sommer, S., A. Toto Volahy, and U.S. Seal 'A population and habitat viability assessment for the highly endangered giant jumping rat (Hypogeomys antimena), the largest extant endemic rodent of Madagascar', *Animal Conservation* 5 (2002), 263–273.

Star, Susan Leigh. 'The Ethnography of infrastructure', *The American Behavioral Scientist* 43 (3) (1999), 377–391.

Thiessen, Del, and Kent Maxwell 'A glass rodent enclosure: Gerbil city', *Behavior Research Methods & Instrumentation* 11 (6) (1979), 535–537.

Tollenaere, Charlotte, Carine Brouat, Jean-Marc Duplantier, Lila Rahalison, Soanadrasana Rahelinirina, Michel Pascal, Hélène Moné Gabriel Mouahid, Herwig Leirs, Jean-François Cosson, and Brett Riddle 'Phylogeography of the introduced species *Rattus rattus* in the western Indian Ocean, with special emphasis on the colonization history of Madagascar', *Journal of Biogeography* 37 (3) (2010), 398–410.

Vogler, Amy J.,Voahangy Andrianaivoarimanana, Sandra Telfer, Carina M. Hall, Jason W. Sahl, Crystal M. Hepp, Heather Centner, Genevieve Andersen, Dawn N. Birdsell, Lila Rahalison, Roxanne Nottingham, Paul Keim, David M. Wagner, and Minoarisoa Rajerison 'Temporal phylogeography of *Yersinia pestis* in Madagascar: Insights into the long-term maintenance of plague', *PLoS Neglected Tropical Diseases* 11 (9) (2017), e0005887.

von Schitzler, Antina 'Traveling technologies: Infrastructure, ethical regimes, and the materiality of politics in South Africa', *Cultural Anthropology* 28 (4) (2013), 670–693. https://doi.org/10.1111/cuan.12032

Wilschut, Liesbeth I., Elisabeth A. Addink, Hans Heesterbeek, Lise Heier, Anne Laudisoit, Mike Begon, Stephen Davis, Vladimir M. Dubyanksiy, Leonid A. Burdelov and Steven M. de Jong 'Potential corridors and barriers for plague spread in Central Asia', *International Journal of Health Geographics* 12 (49) (2013). DOI:10.1186/1476–072X-12–49

Wilschut, Liesbeth I., Anne Laudisoit, Nelika K. Hughes, Elisabeth A. Addink, Steeven M. de Jong, Hans A. P. Heesterbeek, Jonas Reijniers, Sally Eagle, Vladimir M. Dubyanskiy, and Mike Begon 'Spatial distribution patterns of plague hosts: Point pattern analysis of the burrows of great gerbils in Kazakhstan', *Journal of Biogeography* 42 (2015), 1281–1292.

World Health Organization 'Plague-Madagascar: Disease outbreak news' (November 17, 2017). www.who.int/csr/don/27-november-2017-plague-madagascar/en/

Zeppelini, Caio Graco, Alzira Maria Paiva de Almeida, and Pedro Cordeiro-Estrela 'Zoonosis as ecological entities: A case review of plague', *PLoS Neglected Tropical Diseases* 10 (10) (2016), e0004949.

7 Complexity, anthropology, and epidemics

Hannah Brown

It is late in the evening. The tables around the poolside of an upmarket hotel in Bo, Sierra Leone's second-largest city, host people of many different nationalities. The driveway is jam-packed with four-wheel drive vehicles parked tightly together, each marked with familiar branding; World Health Organisation; UK AID; US AID; Red Cross; Centres for Disease Control. A North American man is joking about how important he finds the evening poolside meals for understanding what is going on in other sectors of the response, as he catches up with staff from the World Health Organisation. There is an eerie intensity to this meeting of professional aid workers, medical staff, and emergency responders that is augmented by the incongruently pleasant surroundings. Outside the large metal gates of the hotel compound, we are hopeful that the Ebola epidemic has peaked, but there are still many new cases in the District each day. There are rumours that the government representatives who read out the daily updates on the radio are under-reporting the scale of the epidemic when they list the number of deaths, and the outbreak appears to be moving into previously unaffected areas of the country.

It is noticeable that staff who work in the Ebola holding centre at Bo Government Hospital have been absent all evening. My colleague explains that they are in a meeting, working on refining the Standard Operating Plan for the centre. Standard operating plans give health workers procedural rules for their work, for example, they describe when and how to use different items of Personal Protective Equipment (PPE) including gloves, marks, and body bags; how often to check patients; and how long to stay inside the treatment area. It is after 10 pm. Someone comments of the doctor in charge, 'He is always like this, he works for hours every day and then spends the evenings working on improving procedures'. Meanwhile, my dinner companion and I talk about a new mobile phone reporting system for infectious disease symptoms that he has been involved in developing, and the various new iterations it is going through.

Designs for different kinds of Ebola treatment facilities and other kinds of intervention were refined significantly during the 2014–16 West African epidemic. These design practices often took place through ongoing reflexive processes undertaken by people embedded within the organisational structures of the response (e.g. Sanchez Carrera 2015). Emerging designs for Ebola management were dependent not only on individual commitment and dedication, but also on many hours of time spent working in these settings, participating in the delivery of services, observing the

DOI: 10.4324/9780429461897-8

work of others, producing and trying out new forms for organisation. In this sense, the work that the staff from the Ebola holding centre were doing that night had much in common with the practices of ethnographic fieldwork.

***

Epidemics are complicated. Their successful management requires an understanding of this complexity. In twenty-first-century disease control, this much, at least, seems to be clear. Public health professionals develop strategies to 'nudge' people into adopting healthy or other desired behaviours within complex worlds (Thaler and Sunstein 2008). Disease control specialists like those in the opening vignette refine ever more complex 'Standard Operating Plans', their expertise embedded in a nuanced understanding of the relative likelihood that risk will unfold in a given situation, combined with optimism about the resilience of solid infrastructures characterised by careful, organised processes. Their models seek to predict who might come into contact with whom, and to intervene upon elaborate socio-technical-material networks that can produce conditions for the spread of pathogens (e.g. see Keck and Lachenal, this volume; Caduff 2015; Kosoy 2018).

Complexity is also an organising concept for contemporary anthropology. Post-modernist conceptualisations of complexity, multiplicity, and hybridity have become central to the anthropological project of the last 25 years and are a key conceptual artefact of anthropological thinking (e.g. see Talia 2017). Understandings of the experience of modernity across the social sciences have become characterised by a dominant motif; the complex interplay and intersection of multiple scales, practices, and actors in the constitution of social worlds. Social practice, identities, and processes are seen as embedded in diverse connections that are shaped by human relationships within deep and shallow time, through proximate and distant space, and through the contingent meeting points between the relational, institutional, political economic, and the personal.

Biomedical and anthropological understandings of complexity are similar. But they are not the same. Drawing upon long-term ethnographic fieldwork in two epidemic contexts (the HIV epidemic in East Africa and the Ebola epidemic in West Africa), this chapter explores what ontologies of complexity in disease control and in anthropology have come to have in common, the ways they are different, and what might be revealed by the dissonances between these different kinds of knowledge.

The general argument is as follows: Over the last twenty years a model of complexity that started out in philosophy and the social sciences (e.g. see Deleuze and Guattari 1987) has become hegemonic beyond social science disciplines, including in spheres of medicine and epidemic management. In other words, disease control experts have started to think more like anthropologists. In particular, there is an increasing recognition among people engaged in epidemic control and public health, of the complex networks in which people live, work, and act as social beings. This includes an increased sensitivity to the ways in which social actions are shaped by broader structural factors such as politics, economics, and history, as well as growing recognition that people do not inhabit singular identity categories, but move through the world within shifting, intersecting processes of social identity which in turn inform social practice.

Whilst models of complexity in social sciences and biomedicine have become more similar, there are important places where they differ. One important difference is that anthropologists generally seek to capture nuance and complexity, rendering these visible in their work. On the other hand, disease control often centres on activities that aim to simplify different forms of complexity. For example, in public health and disease control people often work to produce straight-forward guidelines that are assumed to help people navigate through complex worlds. Meanwhile, although the complex checklists and standard operating plans that now characterise many medical interventions may come closer to an anthropological way of seeing the world, there is still a difference between the way in which complexity is imagined in disease control settings and in anthropology. Standard operating plans and checklists developed for disease control tend to assume that all forms of risk and danger can be pre-emptively accounted for, and therefore see complexity is a problem to be dealt with primarily though documentation, organisation, and planning (cf. Scott 1998). Anthropologists also use careful, rigorous methods of documentation, and try to reach conditions of data saturation through processes of comparison and triangulation gained through long-term immersion in the field. But at the same time, as a general rule, anthropologists implicitly work with a model of complexity that assumes there are things that remain beyond what anthropologists can capture with ethnographic methods. There are dimensions of social life that are so complex they are more or less impossible to know. For many anthropologists, the value of ethnographic fieldwork is precisely that through returning our attention again and again, to the lived realities of people's lives, we can become attuned to those things that are at the edges of our understanding. In this way, ethnographic fieldwork allows us to gain a sense of those things that are at the edges of our comprehension. Ethnographic writing opens up attention to the complexities that take place beyond our descriptions of the concrete, and thereby troubles existing conceptualisations of the world around us (Carrithers 2014; 2018).

This chapter argues that the dissonance and gaps between these ways of thinking about complex worlds suggest points at which disease control efforts and anthropology can come together in productive dialogue. Differences in conceptualisations of complexity mark one of the sites in which there is potential for anthropologists to contribute to epidemic response. In particular, anthropological attention to the ways that responses to epidemics unfold on the ground, and the way in which ethnography is attuned to unexpected dimensions of responses to epidemics constitute important sites at which anthropological work can contribute within outbreak response and public health interventions more widely.

HIV/AIDS, Kenya

March 2000. The large signboard outside Siaya Government Hospital had faded a little under the hot Kenyan sun, but the image of a nuclear family was still clear; a man, woman and their two children pictured in the foreground. The message written in English at the bottom of the signboard read, 'Protect your family: Use a condom every time you have sex'.

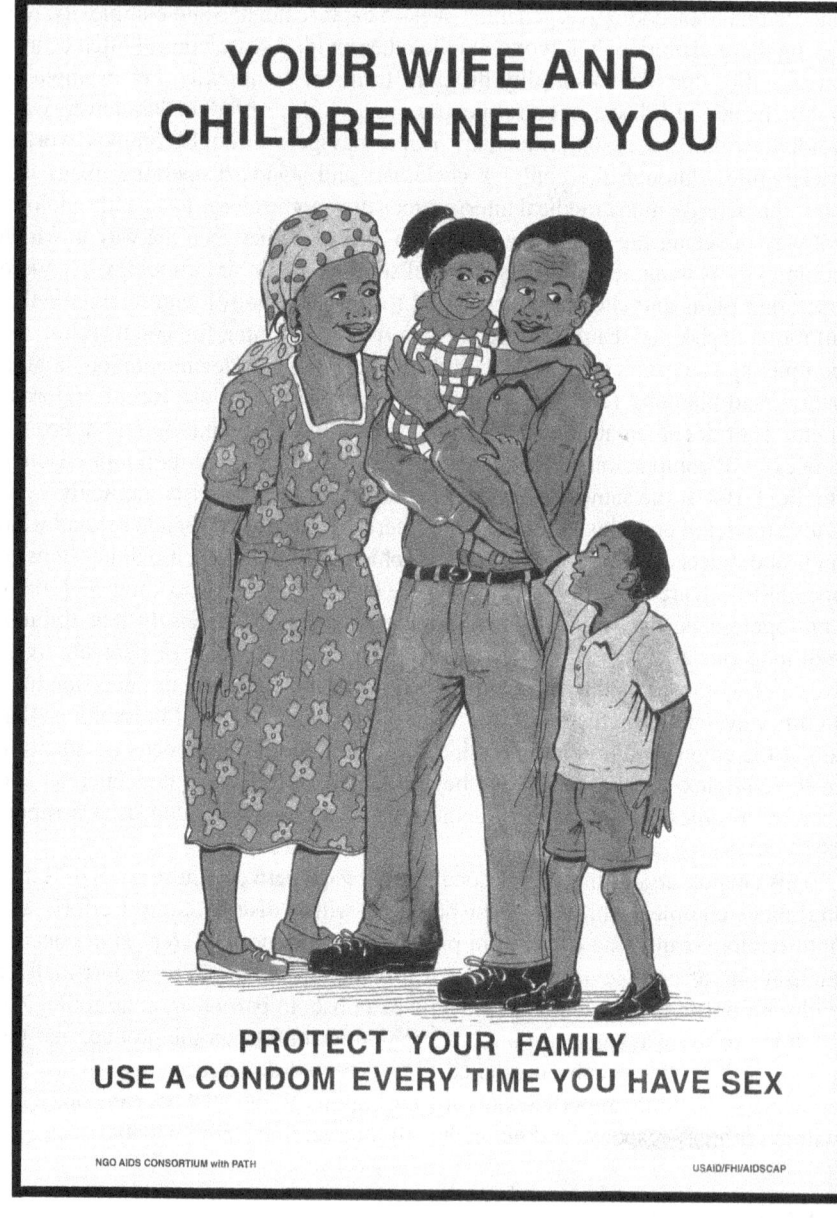

Figure 7.1 AIDS prevention advertisement by the NGO AIDS Consortium with PATH in Kenya.

Credit: Colour lithograph, ca. 1997. WELLCOME Collection

It was five years before the first free HIV medication would be made available in Kenyan government health facilities and, despite the fact that thousands of people in the county were dying slow painful deaths from AIDS, the Kenyan government – like most other African nations at the time – focused its attention on preventing new infections. Since its foundation in the late 1980s, the Kenyan National AIDS Control Programme (NACP) had prioritised establishing a safe blood supply; developing a set of AIDS guidelines for health care professionals; and educating the Kenyan public on modes of transmission. The focus of these preventative strategies was on practises that were understood to put people at risk. Having multiple or extra-marital sexual partners was considered one such 'risk practice' and the signboard at Siaya District Hospital was directed at a form of masculine sexuality assumed to fall within this category of 'risky behaviour', one where men often took sexual partners outside of marriage. The message was clear enough, but in a community where the majority of marriages were polygynous and both men and women generally wanted to have children within these unions, it was hard to see how the advice to men to 'use a condom every time you have sex' mapped onto the more complex reality of people's lives.

As elsewhere in Africa, explanations for HIV prevalence in Western Kenya during the early period of the epidemic leading up to the roll-out of mass treatment often isolated particular 'sexual practices' and 'risk groups' as areas of concern. During the 1980s and 1990s, the realisation that much greater numbers of African women were becoming infected with HIV than was the case in Western Europe and North America prompted a new tranche of studies on 'African sexuality' (e.g. Caldwell et al. 1989) founded on the belief that there must be something about African sexual behaviour that accounted for the epidemiological trends that were visible in sub-Saharan Africa. Some anthropologists described this as framing of the HIV epidemic as the 'invention' of 'African AIDS' (Patton 1990), and criticised the racist underpinnings of these approaches.

The task of unpacking and critiquing ways in which the HIV/AIDS epidemic was being framed in public health and biomedical responses to the disease during the pre-treatment era became an important focus of anthropological research in this period. Anthropologists were among the first to show how the harsh realities of everyday life in contexts of economic insecurity exposed people, especially women, to HIV (e.g. Schoepf 1998). For example, Sandra Wallman's (1996) excellent study of women living in urban Uganda in the early 1990s showed how they endeavoured to secure their own wellbeing and that of their children against very difficult odds. Wallman showed how the economic constraints under which women lived made them more vulnerable than men to contracting HIV/AIDS, even while women were also often blamed for spreading the disease. Similarly, in his influential study on HIV in Haiti, Farmer (1992) showed how 'geographies of blame' intersected with the lived experience of the epidemic, and critiqued the dominant biomedical concept of risk by offering examples of people who became infected without necessarily engaging in 'risky practices' at all. For example, the chapter of his book that documents the life of a woman he calls Anita chronicles the experiences of multiple personal and economic misfortunes that lead her eventually to contract HIV from her single sexual partner. Farmer's ethnography is sufficiently rich that we come to understand that there are many women in Haiti who are like Anita.

Although not strictly speaking written by anthropologists, another contribution to these debates deserves mention here. In 1991 an important article by Randall Packard and Paul Epstein argued that epidemiological discourse about HIV/AIDS was founded on prejudiced ideas about African sexuality.

They wrote,

> [I]t was argued as early as 1985 that the heterosexual transmission of HIV in Africa was the result of higher levels of sexual promiscuity among Africans, or in the current language of social science research on AIDS 'poly-partner sexual activities'. The middle class business-man or bureaucrat with a string of lovers, the truck drivers have sexual contacts all across the African map, and above all the pervasive female prostitute who was said to have literally hundreds of contacts each year, were identified as the main vectors of HIV transmission in Africa.
>
> (1991)

Packard and Epstein argued that there were many reasons why the HIV/AIDS epidemic was following different patterns in sub-Saharan Africa to those seen in other parts of the world. The most significant of these was the political-economic context in which the epidemic was unfolding, but other factors such as the massive re-using of syringes and medical equipment in health facilities were also important. They argued that there was no scientific basis for focusing on sexual behaviour over and above other causes for the spread of the virus, and criticised those social scientists who carried out behavioural research that fell within the paradigm of 'understanding risk practices' rather than exploring the broader question of the different kinds of social conditions that led to the spread of HIV/AIDS. Packard and Epstein argued that this closure of research questions was likely to limit our ability to understand and respond to the epidemic, and that because risk factors were seen as being culturally determined this meant that responders could then blame the spread of HIV/AIDS on the risky practices of those perceived to be spreading the virus, and could ignore significant structural and economic problems that created conditions of risk.

In all of these examples, and many others from this period, the role that anthropologists took in the early part of the HIV/AIDS epidemic was largely to question the terms by which the epidemic was being framed, and push for a deeper and *more complex* understanding of the ways in which people lived, and particularly how forms of economic inequality shaped landscapes of risk. Many anthropologists at the time understood their work on HIV as situated within a critical project that aimed 'to sort out how particular versions of truth are produced and sustained, and what cultural work they do in given contexts' (Treichler 1989: 48). An emergent approach known as Critical Medical Anthropology became a central – some argue defining – orientation within the sub-discipline. Later in the epidemic, with the growing realisation that the risk of contracting HIV was much more widely and complexly distributed than the narrow categories of truck driver/prostitute/ sugar daddy allowed for, and, for example, that one of the strongest markers of risk was being a married heterosexual woman, it was clear how right anthropologists had been to push for a more complex interpretation of risk in terms of the lived nature of the epidemic, and how dangerous the simplification of risk into risk groups had been in terms of public health messaging.

Ebola, Sierra Leone

September 2014. I received an invitation from an epidemiologist colleague to collaborate with a humanitarian non-governmental organisation working in West Africa. Together, we developed a research proposal that combined a short piece of fieldwork on infection prevention control in health facilities that would be followed up with the development of a health-worker-led intervention to be implemented by the NGO (Ratnayake et al. 2016). Two months later, we were ready to start work. It was my first time to travel to an Ebola outbreak and the days before leaving I did what I could to mitigate the fear of travelling to the epicentre of the outbreak at a time when the international media was – literally – at fever pitch. I called a friend who had been working in Guinea and Liberia. She gave me some advice; don't touch anyone or anything; wear covered shoes, not sandals; think about having a bleach spray in your room, so that you can spray the bottoms of your shoes when you get home; have different clothes for 'inside' and 'outside'; don't sit down if you visit health centres or if you go to areas where there are active cases; think about taking your own chair – a plastic one – that you can take with you to the field and spray with bleach afterwards; wash your fruit in water mixed with bleach. Her practical advice reassured me, but I was still worried. My youngest son was six years old. Most nights, I woke to the thud of footsteps on the landing at home as he moved from his bedroom to mine, seeking companionship as he grew frightened by the dark loneliness of the night. Was it safe for me to sleep with and cuddle my child? I wrote to an epidemiologist colleague, who had worked in a number of filo-virus epidemics, for more advice: 'Yes of course it's safe to hug your child. Just stick to the 'no touch' policy when you are away, and avoid large gatherings when you get back, because you don't want to get sick with something and be wondering if it is Ebola'.

These detailed and list-like forms of practical wisdom were the first example I experienced of the importance of what Atul Gawande (2011) calls 'checklists' in the response against Ebola. The checklists I encountered during fieldwork in the period of the epidemic were complex procedures that could be more or less formalised, and which helped people manage situations where they might be at risk. Gawande elaborates his 'checklist manifesto' in a popular book that not only valorises careful list-making, but which also captures the contemporary popularity of the motif of complexity and the ways ideas of complexity have moved beyond anthropology. Drawing on his expertise as a surgeon, Gawande's book considers what he argues is a central problem of modern medicine: the ways in which we have, on the one hand, an increase in medical specialisms and knowledge that has created ever more possibilities for saving lives. On the other hand, we know that mistakes are still made, and that sometimes, the proliferation of multiple technologies and possibilities for action can create further opportunity for error. Gawande's answer to 'The Problem of Extreme Complexity' (this is the title of the opening chapter of the book), is the humble checklist. Checklists are the solution to complex problems, Gawande argues, when they are used to ensure that 'simple steps are not missed or skipped and . . . to make sure that everyone talks through and resolves all the hard and unexpected problems' (2011: 70).

It was whilst doing fieldwork in the Peripheral Health Units of Eastern Sierra Leone, where government health workers were endeavouring to provide routine medical care to pregnant women and sick adults and children and to cope with a situation where people showing symptoms of Ebola might appear seeking care at any time, that I came across a powerful example of the checklist as Gawande imagined it. The seventeen-page document had been produced in September 2014 at the height of the epidemic in Sierra Leone. Entitled, 'Infection control and screening and isolation of suspected Ebola cases at the peripheral units', the document included general guidance for medical practice in the health facility, such as, 'Do not use mobile phones or touch personal items with gloved hands', and 'Minimize unnecessary touching of your face' (Kenema District Health Team et al. 2014: 4). The document went on to explain how to screen patients who arrived at the health facility in order to identify patients suspected of having Ebola before going on to describe how to set up an isolation area and manage suspect patients, and how to organise flows of patients and waste in the health facilities.

When reading the document, and discussing the processes involved with the NGO staff who were using it to train health workers, what was striking was the extraordinary attention to detail and spatial organisation that was included, covering the degree of distance that health workers should keep from patients and their co-workers (1 metre of 'social distance') and down to the position of chairs in the screening area, which should be turned at 90° from the health worker doing the screening, to avoid a situation where the patient vomited and droplets sprayed over the health worker sat opposite them. Written by senior Sierra Leonean health workers who had been at the frontline during the early part of the epidemic in the country, in collaboration with staff from the World Health Organisation and other NGOs with long-term experience working in the country, the document seemed to be informed by an ethnographic sense of working conditions in the health facilities and the ways in which patients and their families might respond to the ways that care and treatment were being organised during the epidemic. In the context of a health system where there were widespread shortages of equipment and resources and families were accustomed to providing many items required for patient care from home, the following passage struck me as being particularly well-tuned to an ethnographic reality of providing care in these settings:

> There should be no upholstered material in . . . [the isolation unit] . . . (e.g., covered furniture, rugs, mattresses) as these are difficult to disinfect.

If there is to be any area for patient sleeping, it must not have a mattress that could absorb infectious fluids. If the families want to provide bedding, this is acceptable however it must be disposed of (burned) after patient departure.

(2014: x)

This section of the document appeared to be underwritten by an awareness of the ways that people often make-do with available equipment (such as upholstered chairs) when they work in settings where basic supplies are not available, as well as a sensistivity towards the kinds of support that families might want to provide their loved ones and the value of the material objects that constituted this support. The implication in this passage, as I interpret it, is that family members should be told in advance that they will not be able to keep any of material comforts that they provide once they leave the isolation unit in an effort to avoid further distress when valuable objects are destroyed.

Billboards

Of course, not all aspects of the Ebola response were characterised by such sensi-tivity to the complexities of the ways that people lived their lives, or such thought-fulness about how people might respond to the management of the outbreak. The public health messages that were visible on billboards and the walls of public buildings, shops, and offices all over Sierra Leone during the epidemic aimed to do something different. These communications were also framed as practical guidance for staying safe during the outbreak, but were presented in much more simple terms, most commonly as lists of dos and don'ts to guide people through the challenge of living in the epidemic.

It is difficult to conceive of a public health emergency that is not accompanied by large-scale health promotion campaigns. The widespread visibility of post-ers, painted messages, and billboards with photographs of leading Sierra Leonean health workers depicted as heroes of the response, particularly in urban areas, did much to visibly increase the profile and sense of presence of the disease during the period of the epidemic. However, anthropologists reflecting on the impact of these messaging campaigns have revealed the ways that these simple guidelines often failed to provide the kinds of practical wisdom or information that people needed when faced, for example, with the challenge of caring for someone who was sick. For example, Sharon Abramovich wrote the following about affected communities in urban Liberia,

'Community leaders sought training to address the following key technical challenges in Ebola management:

- How to properly care for sick people
- How to isolate sick people
- How to manage quarantines safely
- How to administer community-based holding centres
- How to transport sick people safely

- How to isolate corpses
- How to bury infected corpses when corpse removal teams did not come
- How to maintain personal and household hygiene and use hygiene materials
- How to make use of available PPE
- How to properly disinfect their homes.

Notably, they were not seeking the basic information about Ebola then offered during health communications campaigns (ex. "What is Ebola? Have you ever heard of Ebola?") (Abramowitz et al. 2015: 8).

Similarly, Paul Richards (2016) argues that at the beginning of the epidemic, too much emphasis was placed on public health messaging. Whilst it was important to provide people with information about Ebola, he argues that the information was sometimes incorrect, thereby undermining people's confidence in health authorities and that responders didn't pay enough attention to the kinds of responses that affected communities were developing to protect themselves, refusing to recognise the importance of what he terms 'people's epidemiology'. Like Abramowicz, Richards describes people demanding practical advice – for example, how to safely give water to a patient or care for a sick child whilst waiting for the ambulance to arrive.

Similarly, in work I have carried out with Jesse Bonwitt and others, we have shown how bans on hunting and eating 'bushmeat' were problematic both from a public health perspective (as there was probably only one case of animal to human transmission of the virus during the whole epidemic) and also because the ban didn't chime with people's own experiences of risk (Bonwitt et al. 2018). Many people had eaten meat from wild animals for years without incident and found it hard to believe that bushmeat consumption was implicated in the spread of the epidemic. Meanwhile, this meat constituted an important – and cheap – source of protein in people's diets. The contradictions that existed between the messaging and people's own experiences of bushmeat consumption in communities that were also suffering economic and social hardship because of the epidemic caused the trade in wild meat to be pushed underground. This rendered the development of acceptable forms of disease surveillance in animal populations impossible, and created a sense of wider distrust in public health messages.

Anthropologists

While the public health advertising that appeared during the outbreak might have drawn upon familiar strategies of simplification, the epidemic response also enrolled anthropologists in ways not previously seen. Barrie and Bonnie Hewlett had laid the groundwork for anthropological involvement in Ebola response in their work in Uganda and the DRC (Hewlett and Hewlett 2008), but anthropologists played a role in the West Africa outbreak that was unprecedented. Three networks were developed 'to disseminate information, inform policy, and mobilize political activism around the epidemic response' (Abramowitz 2017), including the Ebola Response Anthropology Platform, whose members worked to provide social science resources to policy makers during the epidemic and produced extensive briefing materials and advice on how to develop locally appropriate interventions through the period of the response.

It is pertinent to the argument of this chapter that anthropological knowledge was sought out, required, and valued to such a great extent at this time. For example, responders wanted to understand how people prepared bodies and buried their dead (e.g. Richards 2016), and searched for anthropologists who could provide this information. The increased reliance on anthological approaches is evidenced by the resources provided to support anthropological networks, the embedding of anthropologists in certain aspects of the response such as the building of treatment centres, and the use of anthropologists to explore the reasons behind issues of 'resistance' or 'reticence' to public health messaging (e.g. Anoko 2014). Whilst the contribution of anthropologists was small in comparison to that of other fields of response, particularly in financial terms (Abramowitz 2017), the 'concept of "anthropology" came to serve as a semantic marker of solidarity with local populations, respect for customary practices and local sociopolitical realities, and an avowed belief in the capacities of local populations to lead localized epidemic prevention and response efforts (ibid.: 421)'. As Abramovicz argues, the discipline of anthropology went from a position of being a relatively weak outsider in terms of developing the terms of the response to gaining recognition as offering important contributions to outbreak response.

The problem of extreme complexity

The role of anthropology in epidemic contexts has changed considerably since the early part of the HIV epidemic, and, as we have seen in the recent Ebola outbreak, continues to change and develop as anthropologists work more closely with allies in other fields and anthropological responses come to be considered more central components of epidemic control. The broad changes that I have mapped out from the 1990s to the present highlight a shift from a largely 'critical' role for anthropologists who sought to change the terms of the debate to a more collaborative, engaged role that often includes elements of critique but also works beyond this paradigm. This shift is mirrored elsewhere. At the 2018 annual meeting for Anthropology in *Médecins Sans Frontières* (MSF), the organiser described to me the long struggle to make anthropological approaches as part of the mainstream thinking of the organisation. Now that anthropologists are employed more often in MSF, both in field settings and at HQ, the terms of the debate have changed – and the focus has moved to a consideration of how best anthropologists can contribute, and to thinking about the merits of different modes of collaboration and engagement. In this chapter, I have argued that these shifts in the way that anthropology is being enrolled in epidemic responses is partly due to a change in ways of thinking about epidemics, and, in particular, because an understanding of complexity that started off in the social sciences and was popularised in anthropological reflections on the HIV epidemic is now increasingly shared by biomedical practitioners who recognise its value in outbreak response settings.

Returning to the development of Standard Operating Plans in health settings in epidemic contexts, I want to suggest that these interventions not only highlight a recognition of complexity but also reveal places where biomedical understandings of complexity reaches their limits. Personal protective equipment such as gloves, gowns, and goggles, works well at stopping the spread of infection because its proper use entails recognition of social multiplicity and complexity, and the many different ways in which human lives and material objects shape, affect, and interact with each other. PPE is what we might want to think of as a post-modern object, embedded in multiple relations and designed to be used in ways that are cognisant of the complex, networked social worlds in which people live. If we think about the quite different jobs that boots, gloves, goggles, face-shields, and other items of protective equipment are expected to do, or consider the complex rules for putting on and taking off protective materials, the use of PPE in hospital settings reveals a sensitivity to the very complex multivalent relationships within which it is used. But PPE also works on the assumption that it is possible to tease apart people's entanglements with the world into a more straightforward network of relations and interactions. In a sense, the use of protective equipment in health settings is an attempt to render the postmodern modern, to return complex networks into more simple meetings and interactions in an effort to produce a world where some things can be separated from other things.

I argued in the opening of this chapter that anthropological fieldwork often tries to keep in mind the ways social complexity can unfold at the limits of what we think we know, and even of what it might be possible for us to know. Anthropology therefore reminds us that we can never take objects out of the social worlds in which they are used and that, in essence, whilst we can do out best to work in complex worlds, we can never fully simplify them. This means that, as in the case of the billboards described previously and the problems that were encountered in the delivery of simple health messages during the Ebola epidemic, we cannot assume that introducing new kinds of protective equipment into health settings is simply a question of giving people access to objects and knowledge about how to use them, or that we can map in advance all the ways in which such equipment will be used, or what they will signify to people who encounter them. We also need to explore and understand how these objects are used in the settings where they are introduced.

A case in point: During the epidemic in Sierra Leone, I visited a health setting that had received training in new infection prevention control measures two days previously. At the gate to the hospital, the staff had set up a screening table. All the items asked for in the protocol were present, including a hand-washing station nearby, a list of screening questions to ask patients who arrived at the station, an infra-red thermometer, and a box of gloves. A nurse dressed in protective equipment sat at the screening station. However, a second woman was sitting on the bench immediately next to the man doing the screening, as it provided a convenient location to open and lower a rope that let vehicles into the health centre and the bench on which the screener was sitting offered a comfortable and shady place to sit. He was protected. Her lack of protection was striking. Meanwhile, only those patients attending the clinic who visibly appeared to be sick were screened; pregnant women walked straight through the screening station for antenatal appointments without having their temperature taken, as did other regular visitors such as a woman who arrived to sell biscuits and sweet soft drinks.

In a more recent example, during a visit to Sierra Leone in 2018, I carried out fieldwork in the maternity ward and the main triage area of Kenema Government Hospital. The hospital had been very badly affected in the Ebola outbreak. The deaths of forty-two hospital staff during the Ebola outbreak were commemorated on a monument at the entrance to compound. They had died partly because of a lack of basic resources like gloves and bleach, especially in the early part of the epidemic. In 2018, the staff I observed were again forced to work without sufficient protective equipment. In this instance the guidelines available (including a copy of a 100-page document available on the nurses' desk in the triage) lacked sufficient or relevant information. If there is no bleach, is it better to wash a stethoscope in 'plain water' (water containing neither soap nor bleach) or to wipe it with a tissue? If gloves are in short supply, is it safe to try and do examinations with one hand, and use only one glove each time, or better to send patients' families to buy gloves outside the hospital, even though this may delay their treatment? If there are no protective gowns available, is it reasonable to ask a patient's family members (who have already been in close contact with the sick person) to carry their patient to a hospital bed for admission? These are the kinds of challenges that the health workers I was observing were dealing with as they carried out their work. Standard Operating Plans for using protective equipment in resource-limited settings need to include suggestions for safe ways of working when these objects are in short supply. And whilst a good plan should be able to pre-empt locally specific challenges that may arise – such as the distress of family members who have to observe the burning of property that belonged to a sick person – anthropology teaches us that we always need to keep in mind the unexpected and complex dimensions of social life that lie at the limits of our conceptualisations of the world and which are revealed in the lived realities of social practice.

References

Abramowitz, Sharon 'Epidemics (Especially Ebola)', *Annual Review of Anthropology* 46 (1) (2017), 421–445.

Abramowitz, Sharon Alane, et al. 'Community-centered responses to Ebola in urban Liberia: The view from below', *PLOS Neglected Tropical Diseases* 9 (4) (2015), e0003706.

Anoko, Julienne N. 'Communication with rebellious communities during an outbreak of Ebola Virus Disease in Guinea: An anthropological approach', *Ebola Response Anthropology Platform* (2014). www.ebola-anthropology.net/case_studies/communication-with-rebellious-communities-during-an-outbreak-of-ebola-virus-disease-in-guinea-an-anthropological-approach/, accessed October 07, 2016.

Bonwitt, Jesse, et al. 'Unintended consequences of the 'bushmeat ban' in West Africa during the 2013–2016 Ebola virus disease epidemic', *Social Science & Medicine* 200 (2018), 166–173.

Caduff, Carlo *The Pandemic Perhaps: Dramatic Events in a Public Culture of Danger* (Berkeley, CA: The University of California Press, 2015).

Caldwell, John C., Pat Caldwell, and Pat Quiggin 'The social context of AIDS in sub-Saharan Africa', *Population and Development Review* 15 (2) (1989), 185–234.

Carrithers, Michael 'Anthropology as irony and philosophy, or the knots in simple ethnographic projects', *HAU: Journal of Ethnographic Theory* 4 (3) (2014), 117–142.

Carrithers, Michael 'How to open a world 1: Humanism as method', In F. Girke (ed.), *Anthropology as Homage* (Cologne: Rüdiger Köppe Verlag, 2018).

Deleuze, Giles, and Felix Guattari Capitalism *and Schizophrenia II: A Thousand Plateaus* (London and New York: Continuum, 1987).

Farmer, Paul *AIDS and Accusation: Haiti and the Geography of Blame* (Berkeley, CA: University of California Press, 1992).

Gawande, Atul *The Checklist Manifesto: How to Get Things Right* (London: Profile Books, 2011).

Hewlett, Barry, and Bonnie Hewlett *Ebola, Culture, and Politics: The Anthropology of an Emerging Disease* (Belmont, CA: Thomson Wadsworth, 2008).

Kenema District Health Team, et al. *Infection Control and Screening and Isolation of Suspected Ebola Cases at the Peripheral Health Units (PHUs): Infection Control Guidelines and Training Manual* (Freetown: Ministry of Health and Sanitation, 2014).

Kosoy, Michael, and Roman Kosoy 'Complexity and biosemiotics in evolutionary ecology of zoonotic infectious agents', *Evolutionary Applications* 11 (4) (2018), 394–403.

Packard, Randall M., and Paul Epstein 'Epidemiologists, social scientists, and the structure of medical research on AIDS in Africa', *Social Science and Medicine* 33 (7) (1991), 771–794.

Patton, Cindy *Inventing AIDS* (New York and London: Routledge, 1990).

Ratnayake, Ruwan, et al. 'Improving Ebola infection prevention and control in primary healthcare facilities in Sierra Leone: A single-group pretest post-test, mixed-methods study', *BMJ Global Health* 1 (4) (2016), 1, e000103.

Richards, Paul *Ebola: How a People's Science Helped end an Epidemic* (London: Zed Books, 2016).

Sanchez Carrera, Verónica. *Ebola Review: Ebola Treatment Centers: Design and Construction. Part I. Evaluation Outcomes* (MSF OCB, 2015). http://cdn.evaluation.msf.org/sites/evaluation/files/attachments/seu_ebola_report_etc_design_and_construction_part_i_final_0.pdf

Schoepf, Brooke Grundfest 'Inscribing the body politic: Women and AIDS in Africa', In M. Lock, and P. Kaufert (eds.), *Pragmatic Women and Body Politics*, pp. 98–126 (Cambridge: Cambridge University Press, 1998).

Scott, James C. *Seeing like a State: How Certain Schemes to Improve the Human Condition Have Failed* (New Haven, CT and London: Yale University Press, 1998).

Talia, Dan-Cohen 'Epistemic artefacts: On the uses of complexity in anthropology', *Journal of the Royal Anthropological Institute* 23 (2) (2017), 285–301.

Thaler, Richard H., and Cass R. Sunstein *Nudge: Improving Decisions about Health, Wealth and Happiness* (New Haven, CT and London: Yale University Press, 2008).

Treichler, Paula 'AIDS and HIV infection in the third world: A first world chronicle', In B. Kruger, and P. Mariani (eds.), *Remaking History*, pp. 377–401 (Seattle: Bay Press, 1989).

Wallman, Sandra, ed. *Kampala Women Getting By: Wellbeing in the Time of AIDS* (London, Kampala and Athens: James Currey, 1996).

8 Pandemic publics

How epidemics transform social and political collectives of public health

Ruth Prince

Introduction

How do epidemics interpellate publics? Epidemics, at least those that gain visibility, focus funding, intervention, expertise, and global attention on a particular disease. They bring specific populations to attention, both in relation to concerns about exposure and efforts at intervention and containment. Historically, epidemic responses have placed in circulation powerful images and judgements of these populations, places, and individuals, for example, as 'unsanitary subjects' (Briggs and Martini-Briggs 2003), calling them into being, one could argue, in terms of public perception and presence. There exists a large literature concerning how colonial and imperial epidemic responses presented colonial subjects as both 'unhygienic' and 'backward', in need of modern medicine and civilisation (Vaughan 1991, 1994; Arnold 1993; Echenberg 2002), but one does not need to rely on historical examples, as the recent Ebola epidemic has underlined. Medical, public health, and scientific responses to epidemics – aimed at prevention, containment, treatment, and care – have also connected such populations to national and global institutions and resources, scientific and public health knowledge and expertise, and biomedical interventions in particular ways. However, the ways in which these connections have been imagined and practiced, and the conceptual frameworks at play – terms such 'publics', 'citizens', 'civil society', 'community' and indeed 'population' – are unclear. In this chapter, I ask what is at stake in the construction of these collectivities. Drawing on the case of HIV/AIDS in Kenya I explore permutations in the social and political collectives that formed around the global response to the epidemic in East Africa. Here, specific populations and groups, brought into focus through flows of global funding and transnational interventions, gathered social visibility and political traction while others faded into the background. I explore tensions between visibility and invisibility, and consider what is at stake in these struggles, both for local moral economies of identity and value and for ambitions surrounding public health as an arena of the public good.

I introduce the term 'pandemic publics' to draw attention to the interplay of visibility and presentation, voice, and audience in the process by which particular collectives are brought into being over the course of an epidemic. The term 'public' is commonly used to denote a distinct social entity, 'characteristic of the

DOI: 10.4324/9780429461897-9

contemporary world, comprising individuals who may or may not ever meet face to face' (Pritchett 2011: 41). Karin Barber argues that publics come into being through being imagined and addressed, and that a public can be imagined to reach out 'beyond the known community to wider populations, whether politically or religiously defined' (2007:139–40). As publics are brought into existence through mediated encounters, the contemporary world is composed of many, overlapping, publics (lately multiplied by social media). Much of the literature on the public sphere, departing from Habermas, explores how publics come into being through the printing press and media, or through religious and other forms of assembly. However, such registers operate among others, and more recent scholarship attends to materials, affects, and sentiments in the formation of publics and the making of identities, and to sites of negotiation or struggle, in which presence and power is claimed through registers of visibility and audibility (Meyer 2011). Publics and 'counterpublics' (Warner 2002) may be urban, gendered, religious, or 'experimental'; they are often emergent or situational (Englund 2011; Kelly and Lezaun 2014; Montgomery and Pool 2017). Several authors have pointed out that the term 'public' is far from clear; as a normative historical specific concept developed by Habermas, it refers both to the public sphere understood as an arena of debate and to a body of individuals participating in these arenas. But it can also refer more generally to 'matters that concern a community as a whole, open to all persons and generally known' (Meyer 2011: 150). The term 'public' is useful, then, because its contours do not map clearly onto territorial forms of belonging such as citizenship, opening up questions about the social and political dynamics of such collectives. In an edited book, *Public Culture and Christianity in Africa*, Harri Englund moves beyond Habermas' focus on deliberative publics to include a recognition of the matters of concern that constitute moral and political publics, and the practices of claim-making that publics engage in (Englund 2011), while retaining a focus on the activity of critical debate.

Publics constitute themselves through dialogue and debate, then, but also through aesthetic styles, material signs, and the performance of particular identities. They not only constitute themselves, they are also imagined by others in ways that may create tension and disagreement. In a piece titled, 'Who Are the Public in Public Health?' Rebecca Marsland (2013) draws upon fieldwork in rural Tanzania to argue that government health officials approach the public as an unruly 'crowd' requiring control and as a 'population' in need of education and intervention. Health officials tried to enact legislation against funeral practices in an attempt to close down debates about arenas of moral uncertainty that surface as 'matters of concern' during funerals. Publics, then, can be acted on as crowds and populations in need of (moral) intervention. However, the publics that come together at assemblies such as funerals have their own ideas about moral responsibility and its relation to collective and individual wellbeing, issues that indeed emerge as 'matters of concern'.

Current global health and development discourses enact a conception of publics more akin to Habermas' view of the public as actors involved in rational-critical debate. Publics are supposed to participate, at the grassroots, in matters that concern them, even while their boundaries are circumscribed within the sphere of 'local communities'. Participation and empowerment have become buzzwords of development. These highly visible 'travelling technologies' exist alongside other imaginaries and practices of the public and other spheres where not only publics are addressed or where people assemble and debate, such as newspapers and literary genres (Barber 2007), but also street parliaments (Banegas and Brisset-Foucault 2012), religious assemblies (Englund 2011), funerals (Durham and Klaits 2002), drinking clubs, and markets. What connects these forms of assembly is not only critical debate but also a focus on claim-making, both in terms of making (moral) claims about oneself and in terms of making claims on others. However, the publics that form in places where people assemble and debate – and their moral, social and political concerns – are often invisible to the actors and institutions operating in the field of global health.

Much has been written about the 'politics of life' surrounding the HIV/AIDS epidemic, including the forms of social and political mobilisation and the emergence of patient groups, civil society activism, and transnational activism (e.g. Epstein 1998; Robbins 2004; Nguyen 2011). Transnational HIV/AIDS activism has certainly brought HIV-positive people and their supporters into being as a new form of transnational public, one that pursues new forms of claim-making and creates new forms of citizenship (e.g. Nguyen 2011). However, critics argue that the focus on a single disease and the celebration of rights in relation to it involve new forms of triage and exclusion and redirects attention away from states' responsibilities for their citizens and from aspirations of 'health for all' (e.g. Mahajan 2012). And while the right-to-treatment movement has had striking success in countries such as South Africa, with its long tradition of anti-apartheid activism, in East African countries the HIV/AIDS epidemic has emerged in very different political and social contexts (Beckmann and Bujra 2010; Marsland 2012; Prince 2012; Whyte et al. 2014). This chapter explores the collectives that have come into being in response to the HIV/AIDs epidemic in East Africa. There is a rich anthropological literature from the early days of AIDS in Africa, which focused on public concerns about moral community, which were often voiced in assemblies such as funerals (e.g. Durham and Klaits 2002; Dilger and Luig 2010; Geissler and Prince 2010a). In this piece, I consider instead the collectivities that are brought into being through policy interventions, and how epidemic interventions assembled a particular imagination of the public. The global health response to the HIV/AIDS epidemic, which grew in force from the early 2000s, reflected a broader development focus on concepts such as participation and empowerment, the grassroots and civil society, and on the organisations tasked with delivering change: NGOs and community-based groups, rather than states and citizens. I draw on ethnographic research in Kisumu, Kenya's third largest city, which became a 'hot spot' of global health interventions from the turn of the twenty-first century, largely as a response to the HIV/AIDS epidemic.

Kisumu as an epidemic hotspot

By the time my ethnographic research in Kisumu began, in late 2008, the prominence of the HIV-AIDS epidemic in western Kenya had created a huge influx of
external funds and of non-governmental and transnational organisations which, in
complex partnerships with the Kenyan state, targeted specific diseases, provided
treatment and care, and supported livelihoods of those who were, in the commonly
used phrase, 'infected and affected by HIV'. In line with the broader trend to
participatory and community-driven development, 'community based' and 'self-
help' groups were favoured recipients of grants from charitable, philanthropic, or
donor agencies, as they were imagined as sites where 'responsible' and 'active'
citizens and communities could articulate their own health care and welfare priorities and become participants in health care provision and development work.
They were also imagined as spaces of social transformation – where individuals
become exposed to new knowledge and skills that, it was imagined, 'empower'
them to be active participants in development. Based on nine months of research
in the city of Kisumu in Kenya in 2008–9 and shorter fieldwork trips in 2010 and
2011, I analyse the assumptions underpinning framings of these groups as worthy
recipients of funds and follow the work of such groups and their members to make
themselves visible to state and non-governmental organisations and to the flow
of external funds. In doing so I consider the significance of 'grassroots' groups
as privileged publics in the field of global health and development policy, in and
beyond Kenya, and argue that the focus on 'groups' contributed to the fragmentation of health care and welfare provision, and exacerbated social inequality.

During the 1990s Kisumu emerged as an epicentre of a regional AIDS epidemic, which drew in HIV-related funds and organisations operating prevention
activities, counselling and care and, since 2005, treatment, as well as projects
focusing on 'orphans and vulnerable children', 'income-generation', and 'micro-
credit'. A plethora of organisations conducting research on HIV operated in the
city alongside an official figure of 907 NGOs and 'community-based' groups.
Buzzwords such as participation, empowerment, and capacity-building circulated
in the city, fuelling an epidemic of workshops, seminars, and training courses.
From being a rather sleepy dusty town in the 1990s, its streets trundled by the
occasional NGO four-by-four or government land-rovers, Kisumu streets became
chocked with NGO and research project vehicles and by the private cars of its
thriving middle class, many of whom worked for the NGOs, and who in turn had
stakes in the expanding minibus, auto-rickshaw, and bicycle taxi industry. Mega
supermarkets and shopping centres with internet cafes and cappuccino shops
were built, catering to the middle class and growing numbers of expatriates. All
this created the impression of economic growth and the circulation of wealth,
holding out the promise of entry into a better life for Kisumu's residents (Prince
2012, 2014).

My ethnographic research, which builds upon previous periods of research
in western Kenya, focused on these interventions and their intersections with
broader moral economies of care and survival. This chapter is based mainly on

research conducted among 'community-based groups' operating in the city, with a focus on 'patient support groups' and persons living with HIV that were attached to HIV treatment clinics organised through partnerships between the Ministry of Health and by NGOs. I also draw upon documents produced by government and by NGO bodies.

The 'NGO city': zones of empowerment and development

Martina is a jovial middle-aged woman who has worked as an accountant, sales representative, assistant teacher, and a volunteer and community health officer, the latter attached to NGO and government HIV/AIDS clinics.[1] Her checkered work life is not unusual in this city, where formal employment is longed for but rarely materialises. Even those with some education and abilities to participate in development interventions rarely find themselves in secure employment, and instead combine a bit of business with self-employment, and volunteering in a development organisation in order to gain contacts. Like others in her position, Martina cannily invested whatever she could save from her infrequent earnings into business and property. She has also made use of the connections and knowledge she gained from her work as a community health officer to create her own NGO. In 2010, she and three of her acquaintances, including a nurse and two teachers, invested some funds into setting up an NGO, buying a plot of land and building a 'health centre'. This they did on the outskirts of the city in a neighbourhood that has grown rapidly over the last decade (with the influx of rural migrants and as those with some resources bought land and built rental houses and shops) and that, like other such neighbourhoods, lacks many services such as water supply and reliable electricity, as well as nearby government clinics. She took me to see the plot, which at the time was still a building site, and showed me the plans for a consulting room, a waiting room, and a meeting room. She referred to the project as 'our NGO'; she had already registered the name of the prospective clinic and its location with the government's 'NGO Co-ordination Board', for which she had to open a bank account in the name of the NGO, and pay a registration fee. When I asked how the clinic would operate she launched into details of the staff and 'volunteers' she would recruit, and her concern to target 'vulnerable' and 'affected' people. This, she said, was to be a clinic 'for the poor', meeting what she saw as a considerable need in the surrounding settlements for health care, providing not only HIV counselling and treatment but also health education classes. A nurse would be employed, but, like so many other NGOs and health centres in the city, she expected that it would attract 'volunteers', people who are eager to associate themselves with health work in return for access to training sessions and sometimes, a small remuneration referred to as 'lunch' or 'transport reimbursement'. Like other clinics operated by NGOs in the city, Martina hoped that the health centre would receive funding and medicines from the government and from GAP, the US organisation that channelled funds from PEPFAR (President's Emergency Plan for AIDS Relief) into AIDS treatment in Kenya, and for this purpose she and her partners had hired someone to write a proposal for funding which they intended to submit to PEPFAR. She argued that, once operational, the health centre would become self-supporting, through charging patients a small fee for consultations and medicines from a well-stocked pharmacy. I wondered aloud how this would work out, given that at the time about twenty-four clinics providing HIV tests and treatments were operating in the city – including government and non-governmental sites – which provided these services free of charge. But Martina was not deterred – this was a financial investment that she believed would be self-sustaining – it would provide returns at the same time as providing a service to 'the community'.

This anecdote reveals the extent to which development and health care in the city of Kisumu – and more generally in Kenya – has become tied up with entrepreneurship. According to the dominant ethos of international AIDS and development industry, entrepreneurial individuals like Martina are ideal actors in 'community-driven development'. While many Kenyans who have some capital or ability to access enough credit invest into property, such as rental buildings, small shops, and pharmacies, or into the transport sector, what was interesting about Martina's project was her attempt to carve out a space that straddled both this profit-making sector and that of NGOs' concerns to respond to needs and provide services. In Martina's enterprise, the provision of care is tied to both the development of 'self-help' capacities among the health-centre 'clients' and to 'income-generation'.

The anecdote also gives some insight into why Kisumu is jokingly referred to by residents as an 'NGO city'. The third largest town in Kenya, with an official population of around half a million people, in 2010 Kisumu boasted a staggering official total of 907 NGOs operating in the city or its hinterlands. The majority (790) of these were national and international organisations with headquarters in Nairobi, ranging from global organisations such as World Vision to a whole array of national NGOs set up by Kenyan individuals or organisations run by Church and mission groups, research groups, or universities in the Global North.[2] The remaining 117 were NGOs with headquarters in Kisumu. These included smaller associations formed by local people – either NGOs similar to Martina's or 'self-help' and 'community-based' groups (such as women's groups, widow's groups, youth groups, HIV-positive patient support groups and income-generating groups) that received funds for further development. This figure does not include CBOs and self-help groups that did not have the resources to register as an NGO or to open a bank account. Actual numbers of CBOs in Kisumu are thus likely to be higher. The proportion of these registered NGOs that conducted, or purported to conduct AIDS-related activities in Kisumu is striking. Ninety-one out of the 117 locally registered NGOs included 'HIV' and 'health' in their range of activities. Most, moreover, were remarkably 'multi-sectorial', and apparently included 'welfare', 'children', 'youth', 'micro-credit', and 'nutrition', as well as sometimes 'sanitation' and 'the environment' among their operations.

Such groups have been favoured recipients of grants from foreign funders and donors as they are imagined as sites where 'responsible' and 'active' individuals and communities can articulate their own needs, generate sustainable projects, and become participants in development. Accordingly, they receive funds for activities that range from providing home-based care for AIDS patients, to 'income-generation' and micro-credit, and the care of orphans. Some CBOs, particularly youth groups, set themselves up as sites where international and national NGOs can find volunteers who have close connections with the 'community' and who can implement projects ranging from identifying 'vulnerable' families with orphans for food parcels and school fee support to conducting questionnaires that assess the distribution of psychosocial stress.

However, it is unclear from such figures how many of these groups actually existed and how they operated. Indeed, a closer look at these groups over a period of time reveals remarkable fluctuation in their existence. Some groups appear to exist only in the name and registration in the NGO coordination board's list. Others appear to be very active, conducting a range of activities in several locations. Yet, it is difficult to locate an office or when one does locate it, one finds that it is in fact a tailoring shop. Sometimes the tailor is also the group's 'secretary', and it appears that most members are simply going about their everyday business, while the leader is the person who gets to attend the workshops run by larger NGOs, or 'stakeholder' meetings convened by the government's National AIDS Control Council.

The phenomenon of 'MUNGOs' (My NGOs) as Kenyans call them is well known, and already remarked upon in the mid-1990s during the turn towards strengthening 'civil society' against the politically repressive and patriarchal state apparatus of the Moi government (Ndegwa 1994). In response to structural adjustment and extreme cuts in the health budget, NGOs were already providing over forty percent of health care services in Kenya in the early 1990s (ibid.; see Hearn 1998, 2002). Since the late 1990s, democracy and gender related NGOs have been overtaken by NGOs working on HIV/AIDS and health issues (see previous) – and there has been a proliferation in numbers. Nationally, the number of registered NGOs grew from 500 in 1990 to 5,229 NGOs in 2009 (NGO Coordination Board 2009). Yet, according to the 2009 report by the NGO coordination board, of 5,229 NGOs registered in Kenya, only 1,334 (twenty-two percent) could be found and interviewed in 2007 and 2008. The report raises the issue of sustainability of the NGO sector, when so many groups rely on external funding for their existence and do not seem to be able to convert such funds into future activities. It also points to issues of 'accountability' and 'lack of transparency' (listing the embezzlement of funds, employment of relatives and lack of 'professionalism', see p. 55 of the report). It certainly appears that the formation of associations as NGOs and the creation of 'projects' allows motivated individuals to access resources, networks, and contacts, and distribute these forms of social and economic capital to one's clients or dependents (which may include relatives and friends). In this way 'community-led development' is led by those in the community who are best positioned, and feeds into processes of economic differentiation rather than into poverty alleviation.

The visibility and activity of local NGOs, including CBOs and self-help groups in Kisumu, was (and continues to be) due in large part to the international focus on 'community-based development' and, within HIV/AIDS funding, on supporting so-called grassroots organisations of people 'affected or infected by HIV' as

part of the shift to a multi-sectoral approach to AIDS. While resources are channelled mainly to international NGOs or large national NGOs, with reputations
for 'transparency', a section of funds are reserved for community-based organisations (CBOs), which are considered to be well-placed in 'the community' to
provide services and conduct grassroots work cheaply and effectively. This is part
of a general shift in international development agenda towards the privatisation
and 'NGO-isation' (Hearn 1998) of health care services, in the wake of structural
adjustment programmes and drastic cuts in state provision (see also Kamat 2004).
Since the late 1990s, the government of Kenya, pushed by donors led by the World
Bank, has pursued a policy of directing donor funding to grassroots, community-
based, and self-help groups that organise to address issues associated with HIV
and deliver services; a process that has, if anything, gathered pace with the rise in
US funding for HIV/AIDS from PEPFAR (which dispersed these through subcon-
tracting to companies and to NGOs) (Pfeiffer 2013; Whyte et al. 2013). Through
'competition rounds', CBOs are encouraged to submit proposals for the funding
of particular projects. Pushed by the World Bank, the government's role has been
to 'monitor and facilitate' the involvement of the community-based sector'.

> What has emerged in response to the large sums of money channeled to HIV
> and AIDS is an AIDS business, in which economies of production are shift-
> ing to service economies, and CSOs (Community Service Organizations) are
> established as a means of profit-making activity.
>
> (Harman 2009: 362)

Much criticism has been levelled at the turn to 'community-based development' (see Harman 2009; Boesten 2011; Li 1996), which extends wider criticism of the NGO-turn in development (Hearn 1998, 2002). Recent work on the
'AIDS industry' draws attention to how the rhetoric of 'community participation'
and 'empowerment' channels expectations, rather than sufficient levels of funding, and – like neo-liberal development in general – encourages competition for
scarce resources (Boeston 2011: 782). The 'equality of opportunity to compete'
(Li 2007) benefits those individuals in the 'community' who are most able to
compete, namely the most entrepreneurial groups and individuals. Moreover, it
forces local groups and initiatives to conform to donor expectations and require-
ments regarding the scope of the projects they can propose and their modes of
implementation, as the structure of funding is to account upwards towards donors
rather than to the people, families and localities they serve. As Boesten (2011)
comments, this severely undermines political action and voice (see also Marsland
2012; Prince 2012).

In Kisumu, one has the impression of a proliferation of groups jostling for
space and visibility to the flow of funds and resources. These resources do not
necessarily flow towards areas of greatest need, but, in line with wider 'archi-
pelago' geography of development, 'hop' onto islands of intervention, particular
projects, populations, and spaces that are considered promising (Hearn 1998; Ferguson 2006; Geissler 2013). Consequently, Kisumu is comprised of associations

and individuals that are striving to gain visibility and prove their worth as participants in development – often through offering their free labour as volunteers (Prince 2015; Prince and Brown 2016). In doing so, group members must prove their belonging to and identification with 'the community', at the same time striving to differentiate themselves as responsible actors in, rather than as targets of, development.

As can be seen in the numbers of CBOs that receive external funding, some of them are successful. This holds out the hope of success for others, encouraged by the rhetoric of 'stakeholders' and expectations of participation. Yet applications outnumber resources available and are fiercely competitive. As I demonstrate next, many initiatives fail while others fragment, as conflicts develop over access to limited resources. Moreover, success is premised on particular skills such as the ability to write proposals, to use a computer, to write in English, and to deploy the rhetoric of 'development talk'. Some individuals and groups become adept at this; others know the right people or have some resources with which they can hire professional proposal writers. The effect is thus to fuel social differentiation and distinction. In Kenya, the opportunities seemingly available for ordinary people to access AIDS and development funding has fed into a pre-existing, historically tiered, class positioning based to a large extent on formal education, a distinction between those who are acted upon (the recipients of development) and those who act upon them. Rather than widening the scope of who can participate in development, this allows only those able to demonstrate the entrepreneurial skills and the 'responsibilised' subjectivity (Beckmann and Bujra, 2010), those who can 'walk the walk and talk the talk', into this narrow opening. Moreover, success itself is transient. Community-based groups often lose their membership when funding ceases and members must find other ways to supplement their incomes. Thus, the rhetoric of inclusion conceals the reality of exclusion.

In this field of funding and the 'projectification' of HIV/AIDS (Whyte et al. 2013; Boesten 2011), so-called 'patient support groups' have become especially privileged recipients of funding. I return to this point below. These structures of aid encourage a certain opportunism, as

> poor people living with HIV have to adapt themselves to the expectations of the AID industry, for example by organising themselves in a certain way (community-based, identifiable groups such as women, people living with HIV/AIDS, the elderly) and to participate according to certain principles (voluntarily, accountable to both funders and beneficiaries).
>
> (Boesten 2011)

Here, those who have little access to other forms of income have to make use of HIV, turning what used to be a stigmatised identity, and still is, in many situations (being HIV-positive, being poor) into a virtue.

This underlines that in Kenya, HIV/AIDS has indeed become a 'project' for those living with it (Boesten 2011). However, the language of empowerment and inclusion that surrounds the AIDS industry extends beyond those living positively with the virus and shapes the social and economic and moral field around it. As the virus itself has developed a material and economic value (Prince 2012), HIV has become a language of morality. It draws lines of social and moral distinction as individuals are forced to situate themselves in relation to HIV knowledge and action, to 'speak about' their status and demonstrate their knowledge. However, while the economies that emerge out of the virus appear to shape a field of opportunities, both for acting upon HIV and for self-development, a closer look suggests this field to be more a mirage than a reality.

Embedded, then, in these figures of NGOs that 'operate' but are not easily traceable in the city is another story of development in Kenya and in Kisumu: of the struggle to access resources and make oneself visible to funding flows, through adopting identities and providing narrative and projects that speak to global health and development concerns (such as 'widows' groups, 'PLWHA', 'orphan care' projects, and so on). It is a story of the dynamics of development 'from below', in which individuals and local associations negotiate between registers of visibility and invisibility, 'transparency' and secrecy, speaking and silence, in their attempts to make a living as well as a life with the virus. Attending to these dynamics of inclusion and exclusion, visibility and invisibility, as well as to what people make visible and what they hide, makes the ethnography of groups and associations in Kisumu a rather fraught undertaking.

Next, I follow the work of some CBOs and their members, focusing on the 'patient support groups' that arose in Kisumu after 2008, attached to US-funded HIV/AIDs clinics. I explore the dynamics between donor assumptions about community-based and patient support groups as worthy recipients of funds, and the expectations of group members, as they work to make themselves visible to and worthy of funding. I also consider the wider geographies of entitlement and responsibility (Massey 2004) that are being implemented through AIDS funding. In a geography of development targeted at particular zones, islands, and archipelagos, the groups and associations that can demonstrate their possession of particular attributes (such as belonging to 'the community' or being 'affected or infected by HIV') can be seen as privileged publics whose visibility gives them access to resources and opportunities, albeit in rather precarious ways.

Navigating the NGO city

In Kenya, the roll-out of free antiretroviral medicines (ART) in specially set-up HIV clinics has been funded mainly by PEPFAR. In Kisumu in 2010, ART was provided through twenty-four health centres (referred to as patient support centres), which included dispensaries and three hospitals (one Catholic, the other two government) (there were sixty-four of these throughout Kisumu district). Some clinics belonged to the Ministry of Health, others were NGO, church or mission clinics, some were youth centres and CBOs, and all were populated by international 'partners' who funded various aspects of their operation, for example, the provision of medicines, staff salaries, or training. These partners ranged from large NGOs set up and funded by USAID, to the Kenyan Medical Research

Institute's partnership with the US Center for Disease Control (CDC), to American or British universities such as the University of California at San Francisco (which pursued large clinical trials on, for example, PMTCT or the prophylactic use of antiretrovirals within 'discordant couples' and at the same time set up an NGO that received and distributed much of the PEPFAR funding for HIV/AIDS care and treatment) (see Crane 2013).

These clinics and centres support 'patient support groups', associations of HIV-positive people who come to the clinic for their HIV treatment and care and have been encouraged to use the buildings for their meetings. Several groups may be attached to one centre and some individuals are members of several groups in the city, while getting their treatment and care from one clinic. From 2008 to 2011, together with a research assistant, I followed twenty families with HIV-positive individuals who were attached to various clinics and support groups. We (mostly my research assistant) visited some every fortnight and others every month in their homes and we also accompanied some to their clinic appointments. These families and individuals did not belong to what is known in East Africa as the 'working-class', those in formal employment. Instead, they mainly survived in the informal economy, doing petty trading, building, laundry, hotel work, while some also became 'volunteers' for AIDS-related projects. Our longitudinal perspective gives insights into the process of 'living with HIV' and with anti-retroviral therapy, and particularly into the struggles of individuals to thrive on medication in a situation of economic scarcity. In this context, it was both socially and economically strategic for individuals to join several different patient support, self-help, or community-based groups, particularly as such groups were favoured recipients of development resources in the form of material goods and opportunities to attend workshops and expand social networks. We made contact with individuals and their families through attending these groups but also through attending the clinics and through other acquaintances. This material offers insights into why people join groups as well as into the fluctuations in membership and the struggles to gain access to resources in an urban economy defined by transience and short-term opportunities.

'God Provides' and 'Hope'

The changing fortunes of two patient support groups in the city provide us with insights into the AIDS economy. GENO ('Hope' in Dholuo) is a youth group formed in 1985 by two Catholic missionary fathers, as a Catholic youth group, where Catholic youth can meet for religious activities and, in its own words, serve the community. At the time of fieldwork it had its own website and meeting house, which was attached to a Catholic centre in one of Kisumu's informal settlements, where members had access to an office with electricity and a computer (although electricity supplies are unstable). When I was introduced to the centre in 2008, many of the youth attached to it were not Catholic, although they were, like many Kenyans, active Christians, and felt a strong attachment to the group itself. Most of these young people had secondary school education, spoke English and Kiswahili well, and were hoping to gain experience and access, through volunteering, to further training opportunities and even, they hoped, to employment with an NGO. During this time, GENO housed several projects and activities, including a patient support group that was set up in 2006 as a meeting forum for people living with HIV/AIDS at a time when the Catholic NGO as well as the Ministry of Health and NGOs (all of them receiving funds for HIV treatment activities) were encouraging such support groups. In 2006, GENO received funds from Action Aid, a UK-based charity, for the support of widows and orphans, and began to channel these resources to the members of the group, providing them with a weekly lunch as well as occasional food baskets. Action Aid also provided funds to support children in secondary school and the youth group members worked as volunteers in connecting these funds with vulnerable families, particularly the families of the mainly women who attended the support group. Group membership flourished, as news spread that NGOs were providing PLWHA ('people living with HIV/AIDS') with material support, and those who had discovered their HIV status and were struggling to survive economically became members. GENO's patient support group became very popular until, according to Rose, a young woman who had been a GENO member from its early days and who had been chosen as leader of the support group, she had to insist that members brought their clinic cards with them to weekly meetings to give evidence of their HIV status. GENO itself was thriving in the midst of this activity as Action Aid also began to provide financial support for some of the youth volunteers as well as some of the patient support group members to attend training workshops run by other NGOs in the city on issues such as HIV counselling and prevention work. The certificates given at the end of these workshops were highly valued as they provided evidence of exposure to the language and skills promoted in global health and development interventions (Prince 2014).

However, in 2008 this funding came to an abrupt stop for reasons that remained obscure to the GENO members I talked to. GENO leaders found they could no longer channel support for school uniforms and fees to support group members, and the cooked lunches and food parcels dried up. As resources to support GENO volunteers also dried up, they also drifted to other organisations and activities, and the meeting house went from being full of enthusiastic youth, to being a place where people just hung out without having much to do. For some months, some members were recruited as volunteers for a World Vision project that sent them to conduct questionnaires on 'psychological stresses' in the surrounding mostly poor neighbourhood – but they received little remuneration for this and became quite disillusioned. As for the patient support group, membership declined, as members pursued their connections to other, more successful patient support groups in the city. Most of the members were single women who already had children and were either widows or separated from their husbands. They lived in single rooms without water or electricity, hastily erected by landlords and rented for around 500 shillings ($5–7 dollars) per month, and they survived by selling vegetables or making and selling fried foods in the neighbourhood. While the patient support group had been imagined as a 'speaking therapy' (see Nguyen 2011), once members found that simply talking about their problems did not bring them any material support, there was little enthusiasm for continuing. People were busy, they had to make some money to feed their families, and a speaking therapy group did not support these concerns. Meetings did continue – members 'sharing' their worries about feeding families, teenage children, school fees and income and medical expenses, as well as side-effects of anti-retroviral therapy, but I noticed that these seemed to have been stimulated by my own interest in the group (and to expectations that I had access to NGOs).

The decline in the fortunes of GENO's support group reflected a trend in access to resources for PLWHA in Kisumu. In the first half of the 2000s NGOs and the government tried to encourage people living with the virus to 'speak out' and 'witness', often through providing material support to such groups – sacks of flour, mobile phones, and credit – and taking members for 'training' seminars in HIV-related skills, and giving them loans for 'income-generating activities' and for further training courses. However, as 'speaking out' became more wide-spread, and support group membership rose, resources dwindled and competition for those resources available increased. Funds were no longer given to patient support groups; instead, these groups, like other community-based groups in the city, were encouraged to submit proposals to the National AIDS Control Council's funding rounds for 'community-based' responses to HIV/AIDS (through which NACC distributed funds received from PEPFAR for such purposes). GENO's patient support group had already gone through a serious crisis before I began my research, as the early members who benefited most from the resources and opportunities available were accused by others of 'eating' funds. Membership broke up, as the pioneers landed work as HIV counsellors for NGOs or invested their windfalls into small businesses such as vegetable stalls or even a small shop. Thus by 2008, those left in GENO were people, mostly women, who were relatively new to the group and who had few other options. Rose, the support group leader, was struggling to make an income herself and spent much of her time developing relationships with other NGOs through volunteering. Although she tried to interest micro-credit organisations in the fortunes of the group – for example, she arranged a meeting with the director of one of these micro-credit banks – these initiatives never took off because the group members could not raise adequate funds as a down-payment for opening a bank account, and thus were not judged to be reliable enough.

As the fortunes of GENO's support group declined in 2008–9, those of other groups in the city rose. 'God Provides' is one of several patient support groups attached to a thriving HIV clinic that is run by the Catholic NGO but financed by PEPFAR funds channelled through an NGO set up by a US University. The rising fortunes of God Provides give us insight into the qualities and capacities that determined success in an increasingly competitive funding environment. This group, which was also founded in 2006, had received a few thousand shillings from the Catholic NGO to register itself as a community-based group and thus had a bank account. Like most other groups in the city, it had a tight bureaucratic structure: a chairman (who led the meetings), a secretary (who took minutes), and a treasurer (who kept account of its finances). These three leaders were well-educated – all had secondary education and one was a teacher. It was quite unusual for patient support members to come from the working classes (those with salaries), as most people lucky enough to have formal employment would try to hide an HIV-positive status, nor did they need the material support that those surviving in the informal economy hoped for. However, in this case, all three leaders were very keen to do something about the problems they could see all around them and through the course of several group meetings they decided that their efforts should focus on providing support to families with orphans. In any way, providing support to orphans was what group members were doing anyway as aunts and uncles or grandmothers. Many of the group's members were supporting the children of deceased relatives, and quite a few of these children were, the group leaders explained to me, HIV-positive. After attending a meeting coordinated by the National AIDS Control Council, in which CBOs were invited to submit proposals for what are known as 'income generating activities' and for activities targeting those 'affected and infected by HIV', the treasurer suggested that the group use some of its funds to hire a proposal writer for 3,000 shillings, to write the proposal for them.

God Provides was successful in its funding application, and received, its leader told me, about 50,000 Kenyan shillings (ca US\$ 800–1,000 at the time) to allow 'vulnerable' families (mostly female-headed, widows looking after orphans) to set up income-generating activities – (mostly providing women with some capital to start up small GENO or a vegetable selling business) as well as to buy school uniforms and materials. Other groups whose leaders were not as articulate and computer-savvy, or who were not as well-connected with the NGOs and government officials who hold 'stakeholder' meetings, were not successful in their bids for funding. In a situation in which every group can demonstrate a need, the ability to access funds depends on particular expertise: the ability to write a proposal (or networking skills and financial resources that enable a group to hire a proposal writer) as well as other evidence of a group's reliability, accountability, and efficiency, such as its record-keeping.

The dynamics of visibility and invisibility

In the final section of this chapter, I turn from the vicissitudes of group making to the interest and motivations of individual members and the dynamics of identity in the HIV city. As the previous section argued, being HIV-positive gained material and economic value, with the introduction of funds for PLWHA and NGOs and the AIDS industry's interest in community-based groups, particular involving people 'affected or infected' with the virus. For some people, AIDS became a 'project', but in order to access funds, people had to conform to the expectations of funders and present themselves in identifiable ways (such as women's groups, widow's groups, PLWHA), and make their needs visible through particular registers, such as living with HIV, and to a particular organisation (NGOs and government).

Most members of patient support groups tended to be unemployed and living at or below the poverty line; that is, at the time of the research they were people who had to make use of their HIV identity because they had few other economic options. It is striking, however, that many of the most visible members of these groups were people who either had openly HIV-positive spouses, or were women past reproductive age who had lost or left their husbands – that is, people for whom HIV was no longer a 'spoiled' identity, as they had already weathered the storm. Indeed many of these women had histories of conflicts with in-laws, particularly after the death of husbands, and had been forced to leave their rural homes. They had managed to make a life for themselves as single women in the city through attaching themselves to an HIV clinic and a patient support group. Through opening up such attachments an HIV identity allowed them to construct a certain moral authority and a status as a 'responsible' person, and one, moreover, who can act as a node for others, linking residents up to networks of clinics, NGOs, and other groups.

For others, particularly for young women and young mothers who were either struggling to find or keep a partner and a marriage together, or to have children and gain status, a positive identity was more ambiguous. These women did attend support group meetings, but often only those in a distant part of town, far from their residence and thus from the eyes and ears of their neighbours. Even this strategy was not always successful. Although it has gained the status of a city, Kisumu is still a rather small town; one can walk around it easily, people know each other, and it is difficult to keep secrets. Younger women who became members of support groups were often struggling with decisions about whether to tell their husbands or boyfriends about their status (in AIDS-talk this is called 'disclosure'). In spite of the rhetoric, circulating within AIDS-talk and the lessons they were given in counselling classes about the benefits of disclosure, most people had also heard enough stories, or had personal experience, of its dangers, of men beating their lovers and wives and even throwing them out of the house. Many women concealed the fact that they were taking ARVs; a common discussion in support group meetings concerned where to hide one's ARVs (cooking pots or, for those who had one, kitchen huts were common hiding places, as men did not usually enter them). These younger members of support groups were also the least consistent; most dropped out or attended irregularly as they struggled to look after young children or earn an income while concealing their status from their neighbours and their sexual partners. For these young people, the material benefits that group membership occasionally gave access to were less – or even less – reliable than the material support given by a husband or lover. This underlines, again, that the 'community' and 'beneficiaries' of global health and HIV/AIDS funding and development aid are not an undifferentiated whole.

Epidemics and the publics of public health

How collectivities are brought into being alongside public health interventions has long been a concern of scholars, both in terms of how they are constituted or made to speak, and in terms of the social solidarities that are formed. The architects of mid-twentieth-century welfare states imagined that a national health system would address a national public and foster its affective relationship with the state. The

UK's National Health Service (NHS) is often cited as a cornerstone of the social contract between the state and its citizens as well as among citizens themselves. In *The Gift Relationship*, Richard Titmuss argued that the UK's NHS would foster a sense of social solidarity and the national collective (Titmuss 1997; Harrington 2009). While epidemics have the potential to mobilise forms of claim-making and force governments to address the protection and health of their citizens – and the global story of HIV/AIDS certainly demonstrates this – in the East African case, IMF-directed structural adjustment drastically undermined national health systems, leaving the AIDS epidemic largely to grassroots responses, supported by NGOs. The huge rises in global funding in the 2000s did not change this pattern. Transnational organisations continued working with NGOs and 'community-based groups' while concerns about national health care services and the entitlements of citizens remained out of the picture (Brown 2015). Even though these epidemic publics were imagined to be the building blocks of 'civil society', global health and development interventions were little concerned with citizenship and its entitlements in relation to public health care, instead focusing on the 'empowerment' of individuals and communities to act for their own development.

This focus on groups and the claims they could make in terms of being worthy recipients of AIDS funding and worthy actors in development is at odds with anthropological accounts of forms of 'therapeutic' or 'pharmaceutical' citizenship emerging in contexts where lack of access to AIDS medicines encouraged alliances between activists in the global north and the global south (Nguyen 2011). In Kisumu, the forms of public presence and claim-making that arose in response to AIDS interventions were based on collectivities not rooted in imaginations of citizenship or of global activism. Susan Whyte and her colleagues' description of the Ugandan situation in terms of 'therapeutic clientship' is more relevant as it captures the degree to which access to care was structured through patron-client relationships of reciprocity and dependence, creating an uneven landscape of therapeutic care (Whyte et al. 2014). My material considers how the global flows of HIV/AIDS interventions and resources – which paradoxically focused on 'vulnerable' populations while also encouraging a competition for resources – created a landscape of groups jostling for public presence and visibility. The success of these groups was based on their ability to present themselves in terms that global health organisations and actors could understand. These epidemic interventions, then, have exacerbated inequality and removed the politics of health from the politics of citizenship. They have depoliticised the field of health care, encouraging individuals and groups to make claims based on needs rather than entitlements, to NGOs rather than to their elected governments and to the state.

Acknowledgements

I am deeply grateful to the individuals, families, and groups in Kisumu who appear in this chapter. I am indebted to the University of Maseno's Faculty of Social Science, and particularly to Professor Eric Nyambedha and Philister Madiega, to Biddy Odindo Maulyn Akech, to Pandipieri and its staff, and to staff members of the Ministry of Health and NGOs working in patient support centres in Kisumu. Research was supported by Smuts Research Fellowship and a Mellon Fellowship at the University of Cambridge; by the Max Planck Center for Social Anthropology's research group on 'Biomedicine in Africa', headed by Professor Richard Rottenberg; and by a Wellcome Trust Grant for the study 'Street Level Health Workers and the African City', held at the London School of Hygiene and Tropical Medicine.

Notes

1 Pseudonyms are used to refer to named individuals and local organisations. International NGOs and organisations are referred to by their proper names.
2 Of the 790 NGOs whose headquarters are outside of Kisumu (mostly in Nairobi), 222 are NGOs that describe themselves as 'international' (ranging from World Vision to 'Basic Needs UK in Kenya', 'Youthnet Africa', and 'Malango Orphan Children Centre'). The rest are NGOs describing themselves as 'national', but as the names indicate, the division into international and national is rather arbitrary.

References

Arnold, David *Colonizing the Body: State Medicine and Epidemic Disease in Nineteenth Century India* (Berkeley, CA: The University of California Press, 1993).

Banégas, Richard, and Florence Brisset-Foucault 'Espaces publics de la parole et pratiques de la citoyenneté en Afrique', *Politique Africaines* 127 (2012), 5–20.

Barber, Karin *The Anthropology of Texts, Persons and Publics: Oral and Written Culture in Africa and Beyond* (Cambridge: University of Cambridge Press, 2007).

Beckmann, N., and J. Bujra 'The politics of the queue: The politicization of people living with HIV/AIDS in Tanzania', *Development and Change* 41 (6) (2010), 1041–1064.

Biehl, Joao 'The activist state: Global pharmaceuticals, AIDS and citizenship in Brazil', *Social Text* 22 (3) (2004), 105–132.

Boesten, Jelke 'Navigating the AIDS industry: Being poor and positive in Tanzania', *Development and Change* 42 (3) (2011), 781–803.

Briggs, C. and Martini-Briggs, C. *Stories in the Time of Cholera: Racial Profiling during a Medical Nightmare* (Berkeley: University of California Press, 2003).

Brown, Hannah 'Global health partnerships, governance, and sovereign responsibility in western Kenya'. *American Ethnologist* 42 (2) (2015), 340–355.

Crane, J. T. *Scrambling for Africa: AIDS, Expertise and the Rise of American Global Health Science* (Ithaca, Cornell University Press, 2013).

Dilger, Hans-Joerg, and Ute Luig, eds. *Morality, Hope and Grief: Anthropologies of AIDS in Africa* (Oxford and New York: Berghahn Books, 2010).

Durham, Deborah, and Frederick Klaits 'Funerals and the public space of sentiment in Botswana', *Journal of Southern African Studies* 28 (4) (2002), 777–785.

Echenberg, Myron *Black Death, White Medicine. Bubonic Plague and the Politics of Public Health in Colonial Senegal* (Oxford: James Currey, 2002).

Englund, Harri *Christianity and Public Culture in Africa* (Athens: Ohio University Press, 2011).

Epstein, Steve *Impure Science: AIDS, Activism and the Politics of Knowledge* (Berkeley: University of California Press, 1998).

Ferguson, James *The Antipolitics Machine: Development, Depoliticization and Bureaucratic Power in Lesotho* (Cambridge: Cambridge University Press, 1990).

Ferguson, James *Global Shadows. African in the Neoliberal World Order* (Durham and London, Duke University Press, 2006).

Geissler, P. Wenzel, and Ruth J. Prince *The Land Is Dying. Contingency, Creativity and Conflict in Western Kenya* (Oxford: Berghahn Books, 2010a).

Geissler, P. Wenzel, and Ruth J. Prince 'Order and decomposition: Challenges of touch in a time of death', In Ute Luig, and Hansjörg Dilger (eds.), *Morality, Hope and Grief: Anthropologies of AIDS in Africa* (Oxford: Berghahn Books, 2010b).

Geissler, P. Wenzel 'Stuck in Ruins or Up and Coming? The Shifting Geography of Urban Health Work in Keisumu, Kenya'. *Africa* 83 (4) (2013), 539–560.

Harman, S. 'Fighting HIV and AIDS: Reconfiguring the state?' *Review of African Political Economy* 36 (121) (2009), 353–367.

Harrington, J. 'Visions of Utopia: Markets, medicine and the National Health Service', *Legal Studies* 29 (3) (2009), 376–399.

Hearn, Julie 'The NGO-isation of Kenyan society: USAID and the restructuring of health care', *Review of African Political Economy* 25 (1998), 89–100.

Hearn, Julie 'The "invisible" NGO: US evangelical missions in Kenya', *Journal of Religion in Africa* 32 (1) (2002), 32–60.

Kamat, S. 'The privatization of public interest: Theorizing NGO discourse in a neoliberal era', *Review of International Political Economy* 11 (2004), 155–176.

Kelly, Ann, and Javier Lezaun, 'Urban mosquitoes, situational publics and the pursuit of interspecies separation in Dar-es-Salam', *American Ethnologist* 41 (2014), 368–383.

Li, Tania Murray 'Images of community: Discourse and strategy in property relations', *Development and Change* 27 (3) (1996), 501–527.

Li, Tania Murray *The Will to Improve: Governmentality, Development and the Practice of Politics* (Durham, NC: Duke University Press, 2007).

Mahajan, Manjari 'The right to health as right to treatment: Shifting conceptions of public health', *Social Research* 79 (4) (2012), 819–836.

Marsland, Rebecca '(Bio)sociality and HIV in Tanzania: Finding a living to support a life', *Medical Anthropology Quarterly* 26 (4) (2012), 470–485.

Marsland, Rebecca 'Who are the public in public health: Debating crowds, populations and publics in Tanzania', In Ruth Prince, and Rebecca Marsland (eds.), *Making and Unmaking Public Health in Africa: Ethnographic and Historical Perspectives*, pp. 75–95 (Athens: Ohio University Press, 2013).

Massey, Doreen 'Geographies of responsibility', *Geografiska Annaler: Series B, Human Geography* 86 (1) (2004), 5–18.

Meyer, Brigit 'Going and making public: Pentecostalism and public religion in Ghana', In Harri Englund (ed.), *Christianity and Public Culture in Africa*, pp. 149–166 (Athens: Ohio University Press, 2011).

Montgomery, Catherine, and Robert Pool 'From "trial community" to "experimental publics": How clinical research shapes public participation', *Critical Public Health* 27 (1) (2017), 50–62.

Ndgewa, S. N. 'Civil society and political change in Africa: The case of non-governmental organizations in Kenya', *International Journal of Comparative Sociology* 25 (1–2) (1994), 19–36.

NGO Coordination Board, National Survey of NGOs Report (2009). http://www.ngobureau.or.ke/Publications/ (Downloaded by [University of Oslo] at 01:26 January 18, 2016).

Nguyen, Vinh-Kim *The Republic of Therapy: Triage and Sovereignty in West Africa's Time of AIDS* (Durham, NC: Duke University Press, 2011).

Pfeiffer, James 'The struggle for a public sector: PEPFAR in Mozambique', In J. Biehl and A. Petryna (eds.), *When People Come First: Critical Studies in Global Health*, pp. 166–181 (Princeton, NJ: Princeton University Press, 2013).

Prince, Ruth J. 'HIV and the moral economy of survival in an East African city', *Medical Anthropology Quarterly* 26 (4) (2012), 534–556.

Prince, Ruth J. 'Situating health and the public in Africa', In Prince, Ruth J. and Rebecca Marsland (eds.), *Making and Unmaking Public Health in Africa: Historical and Ethnographic Perspectives*, pp. 1–54 (Athens: Ohio University Press, 2013).

Prince, Ruth J. 'Precarious projects: Conversions of (biomedical) knowledge in an East African city', *Medical Anthropology* 33 (1) (2014), 68–83.

Prince, Ruth J. 'Seeking incorporation: Voluntary labour and the ambiguities of work, identity and social value in contemporary Kenya', *African Studies Review* 58 (2) (2015), 85–109.

Prince, Ruth J. and Hannah Brown *Volunteer Economies: The Politics and Ethics of Volunteer Labour in Africa* (Oxford, New York, Nairobi: James Currey, 2016).

Pritchett, James 'Christian mission stations in South-Central Africa: Eddies in the flow of global culture', In Harri Englund (ed.), *Christianity and Public Culture in Africa*, pp. 27–49 (Athens: Ohio University Press, 2011).

Robbins, Steve ' "Long live Zackie, long live": AIDS activism, science and citizenship after apartheid', *Journal of Southern African Studies* 30 (3) (2004), 651–672.

Titmuss, R. *The Gift Relationship: From Human Blood to Social Policy* (New York: New Books, 1997 [1970]).

Vaughan, Megan *Curing Their Ills: Colonial Power and African Illness* (Stanford, CA: Stanford University Press, 1991).

Vaughan, Megan 'Health and hegemony: Representations of disease and the creation of the colonial subject in Nyasaland', In Dagmar Engels, and Shula Marks (eds.), *Contesting Colonial Hegemony: State and Society in Africa and India*, pp. 173–201 (London: British Academy Press, 1994).

Warner, Michael *Publics and Counter Publics* (New York: Zone Books, 2002).

Whyte, S. R., M. A. Whyte, L. Meinert, and J. Twebaze 'Therapeutic clientship: Belonging in Uganda's mosaic of AIDS projects', In A. Petryna, and J. Biehl (eds.), *When People Come First: Anthropology and Social Innovation in Global Health* (Princeton, NJ: Princeton University Press, 2014).

9 Of what are epidemics the symptom?

Speed, interlinkage, and infrastructure in molecular anthropology

Vinh-Kim Nguyen

Long-term ethnographic fieldwork generates insights into the social context of infectious diseases and their impact and is of critical value in understanding and putting into critical light global discourses and practices even when these are elaborated far from epidemic zones. While the 'social' is most often mobilised to illuminate how practices can trigger epidemics and sustain transmission of infectious agents, in anthropological terms it refers more broadly to the notion that careful description of everyday life can be used to reveal an 'underneath' structured by underlying logics of power and signification. I begin by referring tentatively to that underneath as infrastructure, and explore how this infrastructure is a lively one, both biological and social intertwined.

Infectious diseases, to belabour the obvious, are caused by micro-organisms – bacteria and viruses mainly, but also fungi and prions. However, disease-causing microbes are a tiny majority of a much vaster ecosystem which colonises our bodies and flourishes in the environment. There is growing evidence that the bacterial ecosystems that populate our gut play a key role in mediating our interaction with the outside world, as evidenced by increasing attention to the role of the microbiome in human health. Moreover it has been argued that a significant part of our own genetic make-up is comprised of fossilised genetic fragments from ancestral infections that is passively reproduced as 'junk DNA' alongside our own genes (MacPhail 2010). The genetic archive constituted by the genes of humans and the micro-organisms that colonise them serves as a register for historical events, but also as a historical agent, re-transcribing and reproducing past traces into a lively present. Epidemics are legible in this genetic archive, and specific molecular epidemiological tools are used to decipher the coded traces of past events. Genomes archive layer after layer of biological events that are also social interactions, yet this archive is active – software within hardware that continues to exercise living effects. It is a living infrastructure – both biological and social, and increasingly audible as we examine its traces in the microbiome and as we shall see here in epidemics.

Molecular epidemiology as a cartography of social infrastructure

Molecular epidemiology – specifically, the use of phylogenetic studies (explained in the following) to analyse epidemics by examining changes in microbial

DOI: 10.4324/9780429461897-10

genomes during outbreaks, described in greater detail next – is unique in its ability to detect and track transmission of infectious agents between humans and from other species into humans. This is because these events are archived in microbial genomes. A key argument of this chapter is that molecular epidemiology in effect maps social infrastructure – the underneath of human conviviality – and therefore can be productively brought into dialogue with ethnography which also seeks to illuminate the structures that underlie social life. A second claim is that a dialogue between molecular epidemiology and anthropology can shed light on the human/non-human interface and the 'species barrier' that maintains it.

While microbial genomes bear the trace of these biosocial – and historical – events, dating and location of these events cannot be done with precision because genetic evolution and transmission cannot be followed in real time. Dates are calculated from probabilities which can only be approximations of actual events. Molecular epidemiology and phylogenetic findings therefore require illumination by empirical studies to provide insight into the historical and sociocultural processes that pattern biosocial events.

This chapter examines how dialogue between molecular epidemiology and anthropology has occurred around epidemics – and how these dialogues provide insights that contribute to anthropology itself. Through specific case studies we will explore how confronting molecular and anthropological approaches can illuminate the origins of epidemics and contribute to understanding how they spread. Both molecular epidemiology and anthropology circle around a shared entity: the 'species barrier' that separates humans from non-humans (whether these be hominids or microbes). This boundary is a highly productive one, as its transgression is genetically loquacious, leaving prolific traces in the molecular archive. Paradoxically, however, as one examines these species boundary-crossing events more closely, they suggest that the barrier is in fact highly porous. Indeed, as noted previously, cross-species events may be so frequent as to constitute a significant part of genomes. What might this imply for anthropology, or our understanding of the human?

Anthropology, ethnography, and the 'species barrier'

We start out with a broad view of anthropology, as being the study of the human. Its signature method is ethnography, which seeks to examine human societies and cultures through participant observation, generating both subjective and objective knowledge necessary to fully grasp the nature of society/culture. Equivalence is often assumed between anthropology and ethnography; however, today neither is reducible to the other. For instance, ethnographic methods are increasingly used outside of anthropology to answer specific empirical questions. Sociologists were the first to use ethnographic studies, going back to the classical studies of urban sociology for which the Chicago School became known in the 1920s. Today research methods that rely on collecting data on social phenomena involving the observer are used across the social sciences and, more relevantly for this chapter, in public health, and are often described as 'ethnographic'. These methods are more properly ethnographic when they include a measure of reflexivity; that is, an analysis of the conditions under which observation became possible and how the act of observation (by that observer), and the modes of participation, contributed to shaping the data.

Ethnography is most often used in infectious diseases research to better understand what is driving infection. This has been the case for HIV since the early years of the epidemic in work investigating culture and sexual risk, or more recently for Ebola and the possible role of bushmeat consumption and funeral practices (discussed a bit later in this chapter).

Often because of the urgency surrounding infectious disease outbreaks, little time or effort can be spent pursuing broader anthropological concerns regarding meaning, power, and subjectivity examined using ethnographic methods (Desclaux and Anoko 2017). Classical theories of identity, kinship, and social structure are often seen as too cumbersome and ill-adapted to the more urgent tasks at hand. Significantly, ethnographic research is often carried out by non-anthropologists (who are unlikely to have had theoretical training) and anthropologists are often called upon to do community engagement and mobilisation or help with communication and messaging – for which they are largely not trained (Benton 2017). Anthropology is a basic science for understanding society – much as physics is a basic science for understanding the universe. Asking an anthropologist to engage in health promotion work is akin to asking a physicist to design a building. Despite these caveats, ethnography deployed in epidemics can nonetheless be used to shed light on anthropological concerns. For instance, attempting to implement a prevention campaign for a recalcitrant community can provoke insight into underlying structures of power and meaning.

Anthropologists use ethnography as much to find the question that matters as to perform conceptual work necessary to developing and testing theories. In the latter case, conceptual work is informed by anthropological theories of social relations. Classical theories include those of kinship, symbolism, social structure or identity, and an abiding sense of the distinction between 'nature' and 'culture'. Concerns relating to power, gender, and subjectivity emerged in the 1980s and persist today but have largely remained committed to an ontological division between the material and 'natural' world and the cultural domain and the 'social' world. More recently, however, the nature–culture dyad has begun to unravel, as each is revealed to be interpenetrated by the other. Human biology is not as invariant as previously thought. Evidence of 'local biologies' (i.e. variations in human biology due to geographical and historical factors) has been bolstered by growing acknowledgement that the human genome registers and reacts to environmental influences, and that these changes can be transmitted. Epigenetics, and epigenomics, may herald a neo-Lamarckian era in human biology (Lock and Nguyen 2018). Climate change is the most recent example of how 'nature' has been irreversibly transformed by social forms (i.e. industrialisation/capitalism); as does the increasingly accepted notion of the Anthropocene as a geological era primarily shaped by human activity. As we shall see, the anthropology of infectious diseases is increasingly confronted with biosocial 'looping effects' as epidemics trigger social and biomedical responses that in turn transform the biological substrates of the epidemic itself, these 'subterranean' and interlinked biological and social processes are what I seek to capture with the term insfrastructure.

Sociologists of science and technology have questioned the assumed ontological divide between nature and culture with its assumption that agency can only be exercised by humans. By revealing the agency of non-human actors, this approach invariably decentres the human and joins other philosophical traditions that have sought to move beyond anthropocentric approaches. The revolt against anthropocentrism – and the drive to dominate nature which threatens to destroy the planet as we know it – inadvertently risks reproducing another binary, however: that of human/non-human. To the extent that the notion of what is the human is a central concern of anthropology, a key site of inquiry is therefore the boundary between human and non-human. In biology, and in the study of infectious diseases, this boundary is known as the 'species barrier'. This is defined by the Oxford dictionary as 'The natural mechanisms that prevent a virus or disease from spreading from one species to another', with a species most commonly defined as a group of individuals able to reproduce sexually. HIV and Ebola, discussed below, come from breaches in the species barrier. These events are archived in viral genomes, enabling molecular studies of past historical events, as we shall see.

Microbial basis of epidemics

Epidemics constitute the most tangible evidence of the species barrier. Most disease-causing microbes in humans originate in animal hosts. Epidemics are the result of zoonotic events; that is, when a pathogen crosses the species barrier into humans. The first incursion across the barrier is most likely to trigger an epidemic because at that time human hosts are still virgin territory. The newly arrived microbe thus takes advantage of a largely susceptible human host population and spreads from host to host. Over time, as humans develop immunity through exposure, epidemics wane and ultimately burn themselves out until a new crossover event with a microbe transformed through evolution in its non-human host reservoir begins the cycle anew.

Most epidemics are due to viruses: these micro-organisms are an order of magnitude smaller than bacteria, life pared down to its bare minimum: genetic information wrapped in a protein envelope. In contrast, bacteria are full-fledged cells, loaded down with the full complement of cellular machinery. Viruses are true parasites and need to commandeer living cells (those of host organisms) to reproduce, whereas bacteria are more autonomous. The material differences between organisms condition fundamentally different temporal scales. 'New' bacterial epidemics are rare – bacterial evolution is bogged down by the relative biological complexity of these organisms. Bacteria are biological bureaucracies compared to viruses' agile, pared down agency. As a result, viral genomes offer a relatively easily interpreted genomic archive of epidemic events.

This is because viral epidemics result from mutations which allow them to rapidly colonise human populations who have not yet been able to develop immunity to the modified organisms. Influenza, for instance, constitutes an annual pandemic because as the flu virus sweeps across the globe, originating in the dense human populations of Asia, it mutates so that it is different enough to be able to re-infect every year anew. Viruses need to keep their hosts alive long enough to infect enough other hosts to keep spreading and, ideally, long enough to be re-infected. Viruses that kill all their hosts off quickly are not likely to cause widespread epidemics, as they burn themselves out.

A more viable strategy, if you must kill your host, is to do so very slowly, which guarantees a long enough period of infectiousness to sustain an epidemic. An example of a virus that is too quick is Ebola virus, whereas HIV is a textbook example of a slow virus. The notion of speed we introduce here refers to the quantity over time of different but interrelated phenomena: the rate of viral mutation (itself directly related to the rate of viral replication); and the number of new onward infections produced by each case of viral infection (called the 'basic reproductive rate'). These rates are not constant but vary in fits and starts; bursts of accelerated viral evolution can occur because of changes in host environments or host interactions: such as when a virus jumps into a more receptive host, or when host behaviour leads to greater transmission.

At the most fundamental level, viral speed is expressed as the number of infections generated over time, such that a 'fast' epidemic like Ebola infects many people in a short period of time, compared to a 'slow' epidemic like HIV. Speed is a product of connectivity. Frequent users of urban transit, railway systems, or airlines know that the fastest route from point A to point B is not the shortest one, but the one that takes itineraries served with the highest frequency, ensuring shorter waiting times and mitigating the impact of missed connections. Molecular epidemiology shows that the speed of viral outbreaks is also dependent on network effects, suggesting that speed is a function of infrastructures of connection.

Molecular epidemiology and the origins of HIV

Molecular epidemiology – and more specific its use to perform phylogenetic analyses – provides a new approach to the species barrier and, by extension, to the anthropology of the boundary between human and non-human. Molecular epidemiology is a comparatively young science, but one that has come to play a growing role in understanding epidemics. The term dates to the early 1970s, when it was used to describe the global distribution of different strains of influenza virus (Eybpoosh et al. 2017). Once the ability to sequence the genomes of micro-organisms became harnessed to growing computational power from the mid-1990s onwards it became possible to perform phylogenetic analyses. This allowed the genetic sequences of micro-organisms to be compared to each other. The degree of difference – or divergence – between genomes maps microbial kinship. Just as siblings share a hierarchically closer common parent then cousins, the more two organisms resemble each other, the more recently they must have diverged from a common ancestor. This allows family trees – or phylogenies – of organisms to be constructed, all the way back to a common ancestor, or founder. Random mutations occurring as micro-organisms replicate are the engine of genetic diversity. Mutations which compromise fitness are chokcd off, kept from reproducing, as hostile conditions – such as host immune systems – pick them off. Successful mutants found families and give rise to branches on the genealogical tree.

Molecular phylogenies are increasingly called upon to track the spread of epidemics, illuminate transmission dynamics, and pinpoint epidemic origins (for Ebola see Georges-Courbot 1997, for the earliest example). Assumptions embedded in the construction of molecular family trees (phylogenies) have been called into question. The first is the assumption of homogenous evolutionary time, the so-called 'molecular clock', such that mutations are assumed to occur at a steady rate over time. This is at odds with theories of 'quantum evolution', such that rates of evolution can vary significantly, particularly in times of accelerated environmental change such as those often associated with the emergence of epidemics. Another assumption is that bursts of differentiation that lead to new family lines being founded are associated with specific 'real world' events, such as cross-species transmission known as zoonotic events. These controversies regarding the interpretation of molecular traces benefit from triangulation with historical and ethnographic sources to ascertain their plausibility.

Most epidemics are believed to originate when a micro-organism crosses the species barrier, leaving an animal host reservoir (such as the chimpanzee for HIV's simian ancestor, bats for Ebola virus, chickens or pigs for influenza, civet cats for SARS, camels for MERS, etc.) to infect humans. Zoonotic events are sporadic, occur with variable frequency, and do not always trigger an epidemic. These events are inevitably social as well as biological events, and are therefore ideally suited for medical anthropological inquiry (Keck and Lynteris 2018). When human/animal interactions are dense and sustained, as in the case of poultry and pig farming in South-East Asia, zoonotic events are regular occurrences and add a genetic froth to the genetic pool. Within this broth viruses can crystallise and sweep across the globe, as in the case of the annual influenza epidemic. Bursts of microbial evolution can be interpolated from the microbial family tree, and correlations can be attempted with actual real-world events such as a cross-species transmission, a climactic event, or a shift in host population dynamics.

HIV's most immediate ancestor is simian immunodeficiency virus of chimpanzees (SIVcpz), a retrovirus found in chimpanzees that inhabit the forests of west-central Africa. This observation is based on studies that have sampled retroviruses from humans and monkeys and sequenced key genes taken from them and compared with existing HIV strains, which have been sampled in order to make clear that their most likely common ancestor was not a human virus but SIVcpz. HIV-2, a rarer and less virulent strain found mainly in West Africa, is believed to be descended from an SIV found in the sooty mangabey monkeys that live in West African jungles (SIVsm). SIVcpz is believed to be an ancient virus, as it is found both in the pan troglodytes troglodytes and schweinfurtheii chimpanzee species that diverged from each other thousands of years ago. Thus, HIV, like most other infectious diseases of humans, is a zoonotic epidemic, and chimpanzees were the primate reservoir from which HIV arose (Sharp et al. 2005).

Controversy over using molecular phylogenetic analyses to infer epidemic origins dogged debates around the origins of HIV, which began when a British journalist, Edward Hooper (1999), argued that contaminated batches of oral polio vaccine inadvertently spread the virus in the 1950s. While the hypothesis has since been largely discredited by molecular epidemiologists who instead point to rapid urbanisation, railways, and sex-ratio imbalances that shifted sexual networks (Faria et al. 2014), Hooper's provocative argument triggered a scramble to construct phylogenetic trees of simian viruses – a particularly challenging task given that captive monkeys are not representative of the wild population, and that taking blood samples from wild monkeys is considered unethical. New methods had to be developed to retrieve DNA from their natural habitats by sampling urine and faeces from the jungle floor.

The molecular scramble for monkey viruses began in earnest after the publication of Hooper's book, which garnered widespread media attention. The book argues that mass inoculation of over a million Africans with an experimental oral poliovirus vaccine (OPV) in the 1950s was responsible for contaminating a large number of humans with SIV. According to the OPV theory, this vaccine was contaminated with SIV because some batches were prepared using chimpanzee kidneys as a culture medium. Hooper found that the earliest recorded cases of HIV were geographically clustered in areas where the experimental vaccine had been administered. Poor record-keeping on the part of the vaccine's developers has made it difficult to counter Hooper's assertion. An alternative archive, however was quickly mobilised to adjudicate the historical dispute: monkey genomes.

Hooper's proposed timing (the 1950s) did not match that of phylogenetic analyses, which suggested that the HIV ancestor virus (aptly named the 'Eve' virus) diversified approximately twenty years earlier. However, these molecular studies could not indicate whether this diversification occurred in humans or chimps and they could not, in and of themselves, refute the OPV hypothesis. They implied that OPV would have had to transmit a variety of genetically different strains of HIV. Other arguments against Hooper's hypothesis were also offered. The vaccine's developers have adamantly denied that chimpanzee cells were ever used in the manufacture of the vaccine; furthermore, it appears that even if this had been the case, SIV would not have survived the processes used to develop the vaccine (Lena and Luciw 2001). Finally, the geographic correlation of early AIDS cases with vaccination sites could be due to an 'ecological fallacy': a coincidence explained by the fact that whatever AIDS cases were present at the time were more likely to have been reported by medical dispensaries that were also used to administer the experimental vaccine.

Instead, and more in line with the molecular timing, was the 'natural transfer' theory that hypothesised that humans were contaminated by the chimpanzee virus through routine contact with their bodily fluids, most likely through the butchering and consumption of bushmeat. However, humans and chimpanzees have shared the same habitat for eons, requiring that a historical change must have occurred to explain why HIV emerged at some point during the twentieth century. In the Belgian Congo between World Wars I and II, forced labour practices implemented under colonial rule led to widespread migration and famines and, it is thought, intensified eating of bushmeat. At that time, both French and Belgian Congo were run as concessions, rented out to private companies that ruthlessly exploited native labour to build railroads and extract rubber and timber from the colonies. Epidemics of sleeping sickness, malaria, and other tropical diseases claimed up to a third of the African population of these colonies (Hochschild 2006). Importantly, the natural transfer theory is supported by phylogenetic analyses that identify the period around 1931 as the most likely time the SIV began to diversify. Because diversification is a response to a changed environment, such as a new host, this suggests that the species jump into humans occurred around 1930.

A different theory has been advanced by New York primatologist Preston Marx, in collaboration with Ernest Drucker, an epidemiologist at the Einstein College of Medicine in the Bronx. Marx's research has concentrated on another virus found in monkeys – SIVsm. (Recall that SIVsm appears to be the ancestor of HIV-2, a human retrovirus found in West Africa that is both less infectious than HIV-1 and does not appear to cause as severe disease in humans as does HIV-1.) Marx and his collaborators found that transmission of SIVsm was an extremely unusual occurrence amongst Africans who had SIVsm-infected monkeys as pets despite their being often bitten; the 'natural transfer' rate appeared to be too low to explain an epidemic. Marx, Alcabes, and Drucker (2001) hypothesised that such rare cross-species infections could be amplified by the serial passage of SIV to humans from an original monkey-infected human through the reuse of needles. This is because, when a micro-organism passes from host to host, it is the most aggressive or virulent form that is most likely to be transmitted onwards. Not only would serial passage explain how larger numbers of people could be contaminated given that reuse of needles was commonplace at the time, but it would account for SIV's mutation into a more virulent HIV strain. In addition to widespread anecdotal evidence that the reuse of needles was common throughout Africa in the post-colonial period as late as the late 1980s, Marx and colleagues have collected data showing that the exponential increase in the worldwide use of needles preceded the decrease in the unit price to support their 'reused needles' hypothesis. The reused needles hypothesis has gained ground since Marx and colleagues' earlier work. For instance recent studies have found high rates of Hepatitis C, which is a blood-borne infection, in older adults in Cameroon (Pepin et al. 2010). Hepatitis C is a blood-borne infection mainly transmitted through transfusions – which were exceedingly rare until the 1970s – and reused needles (Strickland 2006). High rates of Hepatitis C suggest that HIV would have been transmitted as well if it was present. That no HIV was detected in older adults is explained by the simple fact that if HIV had indeed been circulating in the population due to the reuse of needles, those infected would likely have all died by the time these studies were done.

HIV is a slow virus. Its strategy to survive despite killing all its hosts is to kill slowly, so that carriers have time to pass on the virus to others through practices that exchange blood and/or genital secretions. It is a slow epidemic, and one that requires socio-technical systems that put into place arrangements for bodily fluids to be exchanged. Fast epidemics spread along different kinds of socio-technical systems and the interlinkages that result, as we will now see. Epidemics fast and slow materialise different configurations of social, technical, and biological inter-linkages: infrastructures partially glimpsed through ethnography and molecular epidemiology.

Ebola: anthropology amidst an epidemic

The Ebola epidemic that coursed through West Africa in 2014 has emerged as a watershed moment for anthropology and infectious diseases. The outbreak was unexpected, surfacing in a part of the world (Guinea, in West Africa) where it had never appeared before, and for the first time striking large urban areas where it initially spread unchecked. Anthropologists owe a significant measure of their growing influence in infectious disease responses and global health more gener-ally to events in 2014. That summer, in Monrovia, Liberia, a doomsday scenario right out of Hollywood played out, with bodies lying unclaimed in the streets and patients dying outside of shuttered hospitals. The response was slow in com-ing: quarantine camps were established as burial and sanitation teams and pre-vention workers were sent out to instruct 'local populations' to be vigilant and report cases. In some areas, the response was met with indifference and even outright hostility: in Womey, Guinea, eight members of an Ebola prevention team were brutally murdered in September 2014. In an increasingly challenging environment, anthropologists were rapidly seen as key to addressing the ongoing epidemic, particularly in the context of growing suspicion, violence, and contin-ued spread of the epidemic (Desclaux and Anoko 2017). Anthropologists could develop and support what came to be called 'social mobilisation' and 'commu-nity engagement': soothe enflamed communities, calm anxious locals, paper over administrative skirmishes.

In this section I will explore, through the lens of my own involvement in the Ebola epidemic, the practicalities of 'doing anthropology' in the midst of an epi-demic and, more broadly, the relationship between anthropology in epidemics and the anthropology of epidemics. Fieldwork engaged in during an outbreak (an anthropology in infectious disease outbreaks), while often dismissed as of little theoretical interest, can serve to illuminate issues of anthropological significance (an anthropology of infectious diseases). Indeed, the added value of anthropol-ogy and infectious diseases is precisely the insights that come from fieldwork in outbreak communities. Discursive analyses of web documents or interviews with decision makers in Geneva or New York can yield interesting insights but may miss out on crucial phenomena not visible in these distant capitals that interlink humans and microbes through material 'hotspots' (Brown and Kelly 2014) them-selves interlinked by infrastructures of biological and social connection.

The urgency of the Ebola epidemic brought to light a marked division of labour in medical anthropology. Field studies were largely conducted by research assis-tants and contractual 'for-hire' anthropologists mainly from the global South. Meanwhile work published in prestigious journals has been mainly authored by salaried anthropologists based in universities and research institutes in the Global North, or their outposts in the Global South. This academic and racialised division of labour (Benton 2017) has been reflected in the tendency for anthropologists of infectious diseases to focus either on discourses and scientific representations or on their need to expose 'structural violence' on behalf of powerless and voiceless populations rather than the actual practices involved in the making of epidemics as embodied, encultured, and materialised events.

Epidemics are always moments of both biological and social crisis. Crises are events that both dissolve and remake the world; as such they offer a privileged vantage point onto the underneath of everyday life and of the taken-for-granted worlds we inhabit and can illuminate fundamental anthropological concerns. Classically, anthropologists have sought to reveal and explain the infrastructure of social life as it is revealed through culture, most often analysed through lens of identity, kinship, exchange and value, power, embodiment. The temporality of epidemics poses challenges to the kind of long-term fieldwork with which classically trained anthropologists are the most familiar. Fieldwork in epidemics however can shed light on infrastructures and temporalities of biological and social interlinkage otherwise not easily accessible.

Ebola in West Africa 2014–16

The massive Ebola outbreak that struck West Africa in 2014–16 is believed to have killed over ten thousand. The virus is exceptionally lethal, and is thought to kill over half of those who become ill. To date there is no specific treatment for the disease, although non-specific treatments (such as intravenous rehydration to prevent renal failure) can reduce deaths. Nor was there at the time an effective vaccine. Remarkably, it now appears that this unprecedented, and unpredicted, epidemic, befitting a science fiction scenario, stemmed from one single event – an event that led the virus to be transmitted from an infected bat to a young boy (cf Baize et al. 2014; Caroll et al. 2015; Gire et al. 2014; Mate et al. 2015).

At the time, in the face of this terrifying, unforeseen, and out-of-control epidemic, one urgent question could only be answered by molecular epidemiologists: namely, was the epidemic the result of an isolated incident, or had the virus somehow mutated and was as a result far more dangerous than previously thought? The need for molecular epidemiological data raised operational and epistemological issues from the get-go. Operationally, highly contagious blood samples had to be drawn from seriously ill patients stricken with Ebola and transported to laboratories with adequate biosecurity and molecular technological capacity in Europe. Molecular epidemiology offered clues, and raised new questions, about how a previously sporadic and rural epidemic that had until then only ventured once outside of West Africa had triggered a massive international epidemic that at one point threatened to spiral out of control.

All the viruses sequenced in this Ebola epidemic share a common ancestor. The phylogenies point back to a single event, perhaps a bat-bite or a mango contaminated with an infected bat's saliva or urine and inadvertently consumed, that would have been responsible for an unprecedented epidemic. How could one, random event trigger an epidemic?

I heard many explanations in the course of fieldwork in the region in 2014–16. All three countries affected by the epidemic are among the poorest in Africa and indeed the world; two have been ravaged by civil wars. Deforestation and ecological changes due to climate change leading to increased bat–human interlinkages were advanced to explain earlier epidemics in Central Africa (Leroy et al. 2004) but have been criticised by anthropologists for ignoring longer historical transformations in the environment (Leach 2014). Reconstruction in the wake of these wars added infrastructure – notably, in Sierra Leone, a network of roads that made previously treacherous journeys a thing of the past, spurring trade and travel. In this line of reasoning, economic growth intensified travel and allowed the infection to spread along social and economic exchange routes – a scenario borne out by my experiences travelling throughout the region in 2015. Molecular studies subsequently showed that viruses travelled along trade and kinship routes. Cases infected with the same strain were found in patients in separate locations linked by road and family ties. In the case of this rapid epidemic, viral speed depended on human speed since the window of opportunity for the virus to spread before killing its host was so short. Asphalt crafted into roads that withstand the rainy season or the Coltan backbones of mobile phones, as well as the social representations and practices of relatedness and care formed the material and symbolic infrastructure of interlinkage materialised in the molecular biology of the Ebola virus.

Missing the epidemic

We now know that the first Ebola patient died in December 2013, but it took another two and a half months to confirm the presence of Ebola. The first alert was raised by the head of the health outpost in a tiny village in Highland Guinea, Méliandou, after five patients died after presenting with diarrhoea. The Ministry of Health sent an investigative team from the capital a few days later, including some experts from Médecins sans Frontières. As patients continued to sicken and fall ill, suspicion was raised that a common pathogen was at work. In mid-March, MSF staff, deeply worried, consulted an infectious disease expert at their headquarters in Geneva who suspected Lassa fever (WHO 2015). This is a severe illness caused by an RNA virus like Ebola which can also cause bleeding and is therefore also classified as a haemorrhagic fever virus. The term, based on the property of these viruses to cause bleeding, is misleading in one important respect: only a minority of those infected actually bleed. The most common symptoms (fever and diarrhoea) moreover are also those of much more common diseases present throughout the region, such as malaria and typhoid.

This initially led to diagnostic confusion. Many early patients who were sick with Ebola were assumed to have malaria or other more common conditions because they were not bleeding, which is probably why the first group of cases were missed. (Seasoned clinicians explained to me that the tell-tale sign of Ebola is, unexpectedly, hiccups that afflict most patients in the final stages of the disease.)

As the number of seriously ill patients increased, and working on a hunch, MSF arranged to have samples flown to Paris for testing at the Pasteur Institute.

A senior French official told me that when the call came through to him in March of 2014 that a sample from Guinea had tested positive for Ebola, he was in the middle of a formal dinner with leading French infectious disease specialists. The diners discussed the finding, and given that Ebola had never been reported from Guinea, turned to the cheese course suspecting that the result was an error. Subsequently, as we now know, multiple samples tested positive and the epidemic could no longer be ignored. However, as the number of cases seemed to fluctuate up and down, and previous epidemics had always burned themselves out, concern was muted. It was not until June, when MSF sounded the alarm that the number of cases threatened to overwhelm their facilities that greater attention began to be paid to the outbreak. The tipping point was the epidemic in Liberia's capital city Monrovia, in the summer of 2014. There the epidemic spread out of control, hospitals were overrun, and patients died waiting to get in. Bodies were left on the street in scenes that shook the director of the US Centres for Disease Control, Thomas Frieden, when he came to visit in August 2014 (Frieden et al. 2014).

The consensus is that Ebola was missed in those first months because of a convergence of factors. An underfunded and rudimentary health care system was ill-equipped to detect any epidemic in a setting where most patients suffer from malaria and other infectious diseases that are difficult to distinguish from Ebola without specialised tests. Diagnostic infrastructure was lacking, and often attributed to the region's poverty and weak states.

Calling in the anthropologists

Understandably, the role of anthropology during the Ebola epidemic was mainly to provide operational advice to the emergency response that gathered speed in late 2014, rather than to offer the insights afforded by deep understanding of local communities afforded by such 'slow research' (Benton 2017).

While anthropologists are justifiably understood to offer unique insights into cultural 'factors' of relevance to combating epidemics – in this case, for instance, burial practices which were rightly thought to play a key role in transmission because they involved mourners touching the still-infectious bodies of the deceased – understanding of these factors emerges from long-term fieldwork which, importantly, allows these factors to be placed in meaningful context. Anthropologists played an important role in elucidating settings where exposures to non-human hosts could occur, leading to a call to extend the realm of the 'social' to include 'interactions between humans and animals and the ways in which people relate to, use, and live with objects', understood as 'hotspots' for human–non-human interlinkages.

When the epidemic struck West Africa, anthropologists were seen as a key element of the response, to help liaise with 'communities', engineer 'culturally appropriate' prevention messages, and eventually give insight into 'cultural practices' that could be inadvertently transmitting the spread. As has often been remarked, anthropologists are called in because 'culture' is seen as a problem, one to which anthropologists are uniquely qualified to develop solutions. Organisations such as MSF and WHO that were the backbone of the Ebola response were hard-pressed to find anthropologists who had deep knowledge of the field – of local 'culture'. (Anthropologists, to the dismay of their more pragmatic colleagues, regularly point out that the assumptions embedded in prevalent notions of culture and community are often out of sync with the fluid nature of social life.) Those that did – the kind of anthropologists who had been able to conduct sustained long-term fieldwork were largely employed as professors in universities that had hired them for their regional expertise. Ironically, their universities barred them from travelling to Ebola affected areas in 2014 because of the perceived risk and, particularly in the case of US universities, concerns around adverse publicity alarming an already skittish American public and eventual liability should anything happen (Benton 2017; Desclaux and Anoko 2017).

Anthropologists were increasingly sought after in the face of local 'resistance' to measures introduced to combat the epidemic. In Guinea, teams mobilised to 'educate' local communities, hygiene teams deployed to ensure safe water and sanitation, and burial teams to dispose of bodies were met with violence; the most notorious incident being the Womey massacre. In addition to informing communication efforts, anthropologists were increasingly expected to help explain and attenuate resistance. Paradoxically, however, anthropologists are not specifically trained in what would today be called community engagement and mobilisation health promotion work, although they can draw on a range of skills honed in fieldwork – diplomacy, intercultural facilitation, mediation, and social networks to name a few – that are useful in this kind of activity.

The time-lag between the first case and the confirmation of the Ebola epidemic raises another, troubling issue, which is that epidemics can spread undetected; an epidemic can only 'exist' once it has been detected. In effect, an anthropology of infectious diseases must be attentive not only to the social drivers of biological emergence and transmission but also to the conditions which allow biological events to be detected and made tangible in situ. Wilkinson (2017) shows how in fact there was a sophisticated reservoir of local knowledge about fevers where she worked in Sierra Leone that was often dismissed even though it could have offered insight into the ecology of febrile illnesses. In the field I was several times confronted with evidence that in fact Ebola had been present, undetected, in the region, for a long time. If this is indeed the case, previous epidemics likely remained because of limited spread in addition to the reasons it took so long to diagnose the 2014 epidemic: limited infrastructure coupled with diagnostic confusion due to semiotic promiscuity (recall that signs and symptoms of Ebola are also those of multiple, other more common conditions that can also be fatal, such as malaria, typhoid, cholera, as well as Lassa fever).

As the epidemic raged in the summer of 2014, a group of us were asked by French medical researchers to assist in the conduct of a clinical trial for an experimental drug that had shown promise in treating the disease.

A promising drug and an emergency experiment

Favipiravir is an antiviral drug initially developed in 2009 by Toyama Chemical (Furuta et al. 2009), a Japanese pharmaceutical firm whose most widely used product is the broad spectrum intravenous antibiotic Tazocin. (Tazocin is an antibiotic often used in the setting of infections due to bacteria resistant to other antibiotics; a global shortage of Tazocin caused by a fire in the unique plant that manufactures a key ingredient for the drug has contributed to global alarm around the threat posed by multi-drug resistant infections (Davis 2017).) The Japanese conglomerate Fujifilm, seeking to establish a beachhead in the pharmaceutical industry, acquired Toyama in 2008, notably because it had a potential anti-influenza drug T-705 in its pipeline. Flu drugs are potentially a lucrative market considering that flu sickens hundreds of millions (if not billions) annually. It was after its acquisition by Fujifilm for 1.45 billion USD that Toyama ramped efforts to test T-705 – now called favipiravir – as a treatment for influenza. While the drug targets the enzyme responsible for replicating the viral genome of influenza, its spectrum of action is broader because it also impairs the enzyme present in other RNA viruses. When the epidemic struck, experiments were hastily conducted to test for the activity of Favipiravir against the Ebola virus. Tests conducted in mouse cells were promising. Toyama scientists by then had begun to reach out to see if there were teams willing to trial the drug in patients, but were concerned about the logistical and ethical risks entailed in testing a drug previously never used in humans in the midst of a dramatic epidemic that was rapidly spiralling out of control. French scientists had heard of the early trials of favipiravir, and contact was made.

French researchers told me that the Japanese were reassured by the reputation of the researchers and the Pasteur Institute with whom some were affiliated; conversely the French researchers found a pharmaceutical partner that was engaged, flexible, and willing to take risks that more established firms would have avoided. Importantly, Toyama was in effect mimicking biotech start-ups eager to raise their profile in capital markets – a strategy that had already earned its acquisition by Fujifilm. 'Gambling' on a high-profile epidemic like Ebola would generate significant publicity and bid up its market value and earn capital for further research and development. Conversely, for the researchers, 'gambling' on an untested drug was a risk worth taking, as at the time the epidemic was thought to be nearly uniformly fatal and finding a treatment would save countless lives. Curves charting the number of cases were taking off nearly vertically, and in September the CDC forecast that without an effective vaccine or drug, and if the trend continued, up to 1,400,000 people could die before the epidemic levelled off. An informal task force came together to develop a clinical trial of favipiravir in consultation with the Guinean government and MSF Belgium, which was running treatment centres in Guinea. It was a bold gamble, given the logistical and ethical challenges to conducting a clinical trial in one of the poorest countries on the planet on patients dying from a terrifying epidemic.

Trial anthropology

It was in this setting that with anthropologists Frédéric Le Marcis from Lyon and Sylvain Faye from Dakar, with EU funding (through Horizon 2020 grant 666092), I assembled a team of anthropologists and field assistants in Guinea who were to accompany the trial by being 'embedded' in the Ebola Treatment Units that were springing up in response to the epidemic. Importantly, our biomedical colleagues were open and even enthusiastic that we seize the opportunity to include the response itself as an object of ethnographic fieldwork. We agreed, in line with Benjamin Paul, one of the founders of Medical Anthropology, writing almost a half century earlier, that to fight the epidemic it was as important to understand the culture of the response as the culture of the targets of intervention. Our central question was how to do science in an emergency, with the understanding that science was as much about procedures, protocols, and material practices as it was about enlisting local populations.

As part of the clinical trial team, relationships and trust were forged with researchers, with patients and their families, and with the surrounding communities. In addition, we hired and trained field assistants in ethnographic techniques – a painstaking effort that involved a crash course in anthropological theory and methods alongside daily fieldwork exercises. We learned quickly that it was key to conduct this work outside the response itself so that we would not be associated with it. This was for different reasons. Being associated with the most visible part of the response – the Land Cruisers, walkie-talkies, and other trappings – meant our informants would tell us what they assumed we would want to hear; it also meant that our field assistants saw themselves more as educators and interveners rather than as listeners and observers.

The urgency at hand meant that we did not have the mandate to probe further into the question of how the virus crossed over into humans from the presumed bat host reservoir, an issue that would have required ethnographic scrutiny. At the time, it was taken for granted that the practice – common in some areas but not in other – of eating bushmeat was to blame. As a result prevention messages focussed on warning against the consumption of bushmeat. More germane was the problem of human-to-human transmission which was widely acknowledged to be most intense in caregiving for the highly infectious ill and mortuary practices for the deceased. At the time we already knew that bodies were highly infectious. The notion that mortuary practices were foci of infection was borne out, subsequently, by molecular studies that demonstrated chains of transmission originating from funerals (Baize et al. 2014; Caroll et al. 2015; Gire et al. 2014; Mate et al. 2015). The resort burial teams clad in the widely pictured hazmat suits called in to dispose of bodies was epidemiologically appropriate but socially insensitive. Little thought was initially given to the broader symbolic and political implications of burial teams sweeping in to dispose of bodies in secret and unmarked graves. Death, at least in biomedical terms, has come to be defined in narrow biological terms that reflect the evolution of biomedical technology (Lock 2001); yet beings continue to exist in social terms even after the cessation of the heartbeat or brain death. It turned out that depriving grieving families of proper burials and memorial sites in some places triggered epidemics of haunting by the souls of the deceased, who wandered in the night untethered by the rituals which would have assured an orderly passage into the spirit world. 'Safe and dignified burials', initially developed in Central Africa with the help of anthropologists (Epelboin 2009) were gradually introduced to reconcile epidemiological and social necessity, but could encounter losses in translation (Moran 2017).

Fieldwork in and through the trial gradually identified three overlapping objects of ethnographic interest. The first were the Ebola Treatment Units themselves, as the quarantine camps were now called. Some of these units never saw any patients, having been set up either too late or in places that never saw an epidemic. In those that did, members of our team were pressed into service to perform clinical and social duties, suiting up for supportive bedside visits to patients, and to serve as go-betweens for their families waiting outside. This work offered valuable insight into how Ebola was experienced by patients and their loved ones as well as into the complex social dynamics at play within treatment teams that brought together expatriates from all over the world and locals into at times a tense and conflictual relationship.

Through this work we engaged with debates in political anthropology around the notion, first articulated by the philosopher Giorgio Agamben himself in dialogue with Carl Schmitt, that camps are 'ground zero' for contemporary political formations; in other words, that modern political orders are founded on the exclusion and 'encampment' of others against whom political order must be established in order to defend society (Agamben 1998; Schmitt 2005). In the Ebola context, encampment was linked to a long history of colonial and post-colonial extraction: labour camps, but also the internment camps of earlier regimes. They shared formal characteristics with the other camps that populate our world today, most notably refugee camps (or in the latest example, camps for migrant children taken from their parents in the USA). But the Ebola Treatment Units also demonstrated an exemplary logic of triage (Lachenal et al. 2014) clearly stated in the aim of segregating probable, suspect, and low risk cases with the goal of isolating those infectious from the general population. Ironically, the general population in this case (Guineans) are people whose lives are 'barely' worth saving in normal times, given the lack of basic health care infrastructure. A two-fold logic is at work here, whereby some lives are worth saving only to the extent that doing so protects others. In this case, Guinean lives are worth saving since they form an epidemiological buffer against Ebola. Strongly put, Ebola made visible a category of the 'living dead', those in suspended animation, isolated from the living so that others could live (Gomez-Temesio and Le Marcis 2017).

A second ethnographic object were the communities that had been affected by Ebola or were thought to be at geographic risk of outbreaks. These included urban and rural sites. Our team members used ethnography to better grasp social and cultural dynamics relevant to the Ebola response, and to identify what kind of community mobilisation strategies could raise awareness of the disease, encourage people to seek appropriate care in case of symptoms, adopt safe burial practices, and understand and accept clinical trials. While this sounds very 'applied' and more akin to community health work, the key difference here was in the use of ethnography. Rather than deploy field assistants with questionnaires, as noted previously we trained sociology students in participant observation, getting them to identify ethnographic questions based on their own personal interest and iterative visits to specific neighbourhood to build trust, deepen observations, and follow interesting and unexpected leads. Analyses of raw ethnographic data was done through writing-up of fieldnotes and crafting of ethnographic vignettes. This work demonstrated a surprising finding: that contrary to expectations it was inaccurate to speak of a 'weak' state in this context. Rather the State was seen as a powerful and predatory entity, in line with historical experience in a resource-rich country where élites were seen as complicit and enriching themselves in the pillage of natural wealth (Caremel, Faye, and Ouedraogo 2017; Gomez-Temesio and Le Marcis 2017). Similar findings were reported by anthropologists in Sierra Leone and Monrovia, lending weight to the notion that the epidemic, the response to it, and the response to the response, rehearse logics of power inherent to the post-colonial state in Africa, and that reading these political logics in terms of normative notions of 'strong' and 'weak' states is in fact misleading (Goguen and Bolten 2017; Moran 2017; Shepler 2017).

In this setting, alternative forms of social solidarity were organised not so much against the State as in mimicry of it and of the humanitarian organisations viewed as its adjuncts, unwittingly rehearsing the state-mimicry of pandemic drills described by Keck and Lachenal in this volume. It became crucial, in this context, for our efforts to work at the grassroots level with trusted local figures who, by definition, were separate existing forms of bureaucratic, NGO, or traditional authority. Charismatic individuals, and to a lesser extent individuals whose social role depended on trust (such as ambulatory bankers) became for us the key nodes through which adherence to efforts to combat Ebola could be secured. Communities had in fact mobilised in response to the epidemic, setting up local burial brigades for instance, but in the vernacular of resistance to the state, which had led in turn to repression. We expended considerable effort to persuade 'responders' to recognise the existence and the legitimacy of local forms of organisation in a troubled political context.

Finally, a third ethnographic object emerged in the form of research conducted around Ebola. We focussed on the challenges involved in conducting a clinical trial in the context of the Ebola emergency, and the solutions attempted in response. As the response ramped up in October and November of 2014, we were witness to a mad 'scramble for Africa' as NGOs, universities, prominent personalities, research agencies, and a curious assortment of therapeutic entrepreneurs descended on Conakry (Le Marcis and Nguyen 2015). Turf battles were legion. At the time, it was believed that the blood of patients who had been cured of Ebola – 'convalescent serum' – would contain anti-Ebola antibodies that might serve as an effective treatment for those who were acutely ill. Many of the initial Ebola patients were themselves health care workers who were infected by caring for others. Those that survived understood the value of their blood, and they helped organise survivor groups who jealously guarded access to their members, knitting survivorship into biomedical kinship. In line with other ethnographic studies of research in Africa, we witnessed the emergence of 'trial communities', a patchwork of social relations stemming from research, animated by historical anxieties around extraction and unequal exchange (Geissler and Molyneux 2011).

The Ebola crisis revealed a logic of extraction visible in representations of vampires and in actual practices of selling blood. This logic of extraction demonstrated the persistence of pre-capitalist forms of value – or moral economies – and the inability, at least until now, for labour (e.g. participation in trials) to be fully commoditised, or for relations of exchange to occur freely. In the scramble to respond to the epidemic, the majority people who gave their time, their labour, and/or their bodily fluids to help the response were not remunerated even though their efforts generated significant value whether in the form of biomedical commodities, cash flows to international agencies and humanitarian organisations, or grants to researchers.

Returning to the questions of origins and spread, and the molecular epidemiology of the clinic, it now becomes clear that the very ability to conduct molecular studies – which required access to and sampling of patients – was itself dependent on an infrastructure of exchange enabled by the epidemic: the humanitarian and research economies that sprang up in the wake of Ebola. What Wilkinson (2017: 391) notes for Lhassa – that

> political economies of knowledge shape the emergence process by determining what is known, by whom, and how, and what is overlooked . . . inquiry into how diseases are known, calibrated, counted, and constructed adds a new dimension to social science perspectives currently being developed on epidemics

applies equally to the molecular epidemiology of Ebola. The exceptional nature of the Ebola epidemic deployed exceptional means which generated remarkable knowledge about this outbreak's origins and spread, leaving unanswered the question of what other epidemics murmured unheard in the background of everyday fevers.

The intersection of clinical and molecular epidemiology

So far we have considered how molecular epidemiology, and phylogenetic analyses, have been used as research tools to generate insight into epidemics, and showed how these are themselves predicated on specific historical configurations that make samples available to the laboratory. To shed light on the mystery of the origins of the HIV, samples had to be obtained from the environment to better characterise the natural reservoir of the virus. Similar studies are under way for Ebola, where the fruit bat is suspected to be the natural host reservoir although this is not known with the certainty it is for HIV and chimpanzees. Ethnographic research, including oral history and consultation of existing archives, has been key to buttressing – or contesting – claims drawn from molecular evidence. What these examples show however is that the picture drawn from molecular studies reflects the broader political economy of knowledge, and that political and economic factors determine which questions need to be answered. Studies that do get funded limited by factors relating to the collecting of samples – timing and access to host organisms.

This is an important observation, as it indicates that the molecular picture is necessarily a partial one since it is never possible to sample the totality of genomes circulating in a given time or place. Even were one able to do so, it would be under laboratory-like circumstances that are far removed from those of the 'real world' where epidemics happen. To put it another way, the kind of society that could sample and monitor infectious agents in real time would be one where there would be unlikely to be unintended epidemics. This points to another important role for ethnography: describing the circumstances under which epidemiologists and biologists are able to work; in effect describing the practical boundary between what can be known and what cannot be known and exploring ethnographically the realm of the epidemiologically unknowable (because inaccessible to epidemiologic methods). Similarly, as we shall see, molecular epidemiology can reveal worlds empirically inaccessible to anthropologists.

Molecular epidemiology can serve as a more comprehensive register when it is used in regular clinical care, drawing samples under more routine circumstances. Molecular epidemiology has intersected routine clinical practice since the early 2000s when analyses of HIV sequences were used to construct phylogenies (family trees) of the virus in the debate over the origins of HIV. Recall how phylogenies were instrumental in adjudicating disputes relating to the origin of this epidemic. Branch-points in family trees identify moments of genetic exuberance (the equivalent to an epidemic of out-marriage in a previously inbred village) that found new populations that appear as bristly clusters in the family trees. By the early 2000s, once genotyping of patients' viruses became routine to detect drug resistance mutations, analysis of viral genomes was used to tailor drug regimens for patients. At the same time, epidemiologists used genome archives to construct phylogenies to inform public health efforts – in effect using samples gathered in routine clinical practice to map outbreaks. Epidemiologists constructed genetic HIV family trees to pinpoint clusters of transmission (visible in the virtual space of the phylogenetic tree) and therefore provide clues as to where transmission might be occurring in real space and time (for a recent example see Ragonnet-Cronin et al. 2018).

Microbial phylogenies map space and time. Space is plotted out in terms of genetic distance, assumed to correspond to real-world geographic and biological distance. Distantly related micro-organisms are unlikely to be found in the same hosts from whom they acquired the infection; they are found in individuals separated by a longer chain of transmission than close relatives, whose more recent common ancestor was not too far back in time and not too far back in terms of transmission. In other words, as a micro-organism moves from host to host, it mutates. Mutations that give the bearer an advantage when they move to hosts whose immune systems are more efficient at killing certain microbial offspring or variants give a survival advantage, establishing a genetic beachhead that gradually spreads throughout the viral population). Genetic sequences archive space and time. Or, alternatively, they are the materialisation of speed: space over time. Faster transmission means more mutations, more change. Speed is sedimented in viral genomes; snapshots of mutation that are stills of ceaseless viral change. Molecular epidemiology, through phylogenetic analyses, charts viral speed and progress. What is amenable to ethnographic investigation are the collective representations – kinship, culture, identity – and the material correlates of speed. These are the infrastructures of connection: transport links, commerce, and the Internet that collectively shape social connectedness.

It is in the case of HIV that molecular diagrams and their ability to map previously invisible social relations have been most used. HIV is sexually transmitted, which makes it complicated to gather information about transmission networks. Reconstituting the social networks along which HIV spreads requires informants to disclose the identities of sexual partners so that their sexual partners can in turn be identified – something which people are often unwilling or unable to do. To research this, prior consent of sexual partners would be required. As a result the information obtained through consent would therefore be unrepresentative of the broader pool of sexual partners and of little scientific interest.

Molecular epidemiology provides another approach. As an epidemiologist once told me, 'viruses don't lie', and molecular methods allow sexual networks to be elucidated as never before. The closer two viruses are (from two patients) the more 'linked' they are – therefore the viruses of two sexual partners are more alike than the viruses of their partners' partners' partners. Molecular epidemiology plots individual viruses sampled from patients by genetic distance, which corresponds to the likelihood that patients are part of the same chain of transmission. Phylogeny recapitulates kinship. Proximity translates into descent. Such studies have been used to identify 'clusters' of transmission; individuals who share a nearly identical virus and therefore most likely acquired it from each other.

Conclusion

In a fascinating and seminal study, a group of sociologists used another method to reveal sexual networks without requiring informants' disclosure of the names of their sexual partners (Bearman et al. 2004). In a suburban Colorado school, investigators used a computerised questionnaire to ask students to identify other students they had had sex with from a list of those attending the high school. The computer programme anonymised their choices and generated a map of the sexual network. The map looks a bit like one would imagine an airline network map – spokes branch out from a series of linked hubs. In the article, the authors refer to this as a 'spanning tree' network, to refer to how tree branches and roots can entangle while trunks line the side of a road. (In this case the trunks are the inter-hub links.) Three findings emerge from this remarkable study. The first, which confirms other studies of sexual networks, but also of other types of linkage such as internet searches, suggests that the 'lucky few' are hyper connected (i.e. have huge numbers of partners), the majority have a much smaller number, and an 'unlucky few' have very little. This corresponds to common sense and indeed the 'normal' distribution found with many naturally occurring phenomena. When translated into a network, however, this logarithmically increases the degree of connection and potential exposure of individuals the closer they get to the 'hubs' of the sexual network. The second relates to the structure of the network. Since choice of sexual partners is not random, the authors tried to identify rules that would predict the structure they found. They found one, which they called 'the yuck factor': partners did not hook up with ex-partners' current partners' former partners. What is striking here is that this is a kinship rule. In Lévi-Straussian terms, this is a rule that generates exogamy. The third is a practical consequence: just by diminishing by a small number the amount of sexual partners, the sexual network disaggregates, isolating hubs from each other. Small changes in a network can make a big change. Molecular epidemiology reveals a similar picture, with bursts of viral evolution suggesting highly efficient transmission hubs ('super spreaders') that push out large numbers of viruses, which then end up languishing in the evolutionary dead-ends of sexual monogamy.

For many years I presented these studies to make a case for social structure, in the sense first advocated by Durkheim. Unlike Lévi-Strauss' view, the formal properties of social structure are neither linguistic nor a property of Mind; they reflect the ontology of connection. Even in what would seem to be the most intimate and individualised sphere – our choice of sexual partners – we appear to obey algorithmic rules, a powerful argument that the social is structured independently of individual volition or agency. A recent paper, however, suggests that the 'yuck factor' rule may actually not be statistically significant (Stadtfeld et al. 2017). That the chains of transmission revealed by molecular epidemiology parallel those revealed through Bearman's seminal study, as well as pioneering work in the ethnography of sexual networks, suggests that both are offering an albeit partial glimpse of underlying biologically and socially interlinked infrastructures of connectivity. In this respect bacteria, in the manner that they exchange genes, are a model, and the rising problem of antibiotic resistance indicates the danger of human interruptions of ages-old genetic conversations; of the dangers of speed (Landecker 2016). The species barrier, the firewall that separates humans from non-humans, is perhaps better thought of not as a firewall, but as a trading zone for genetic information. Ultimately, might not epidemics be the symptom of deeper architectures of genetic intercourse, in which the human is but an epiphenomenon?

References

Agamben, Giorgio *Homo Sacer: Sovereign Power and Bare Life* (Stanford, CA: Stanford University Press, 1998).

Amit, Chitnis, Diana Rawls, and Jim Moore 'Origin of HIV Type 1 in colonial French equatorial Africa?' *AIDS Research and Human Retroviruses* 16 (1) (2000), 5–8.

Apetrei, Christian, J. Becker, M. Metzger, R. Gautam, J. Engle, A. K. Wales, M. Eyong, P. Enyong, M. Sama, B. T. Foley, E. Drucker, and P. A. Marx 'Potential for HIV transmission through unsafe injections', *AIDS* 20 (7) (2006), 1074–1076.

Baize, Sylvain, Delphine Pannetier, Lisa Oestereich, Toni Rieger, Lamine Koivogui, N'Faly Magassouba, Barrè Soropogui et al. 'Emergence of Zaire Ebola virus disease in Guinea', *New England Journal of Medicine* 371 (15) (2014), 1418–1425.

Beale, John, and Florian Horaud 'Polio vaccine and retroviruses', *Philosophical Transactions of the Royal Society of London, Series B* 356 (1410) (2001), 841–844.

Bearman, Peter S., James Moody, and Katherine Stovel 'Chains of affection: The structure of adolescent romantic and sexual networks', *American Journal of Sociology* 110 (2004), 44–91.

Benton, Adia 'Ebola at a distance: A pathographic account of anthropology's relevance', *Anthropology Quarterly* 90 (2) (2017), 495–424.

Brown, Hannah, and Ann Kelly 'Material proximities and hotspots: Toward an anthropology of viral hemorrhagic fevers', *Medical Anthropology Quarterly* 28 (2) (2014), 280–303.

Caremel, Jean-François, Sylvain Landry B. Faye, and Ramatou Ouedraogo 'The "humanitarian" response to the Ebola epidemic in Guinea. Between routines and exceptions', In Michiel Hofman, and Sokhieng Au (eds.), *The Politics of Fear: Médecins Sans Frontières and the West African Ebola Epidemic*, pp. 63–83 (New York: Oxford University Press, 2017).

Caroll, Miles W., David A. Matthews, Julian A. Hiscox, Michael J. Elmore, Georgios Pollakis, Andrew Rambaut, Roger Hewson, et al. 'Temporal and spatial analysis of the 2014–2015 Ebola virus outbreak in West Africa', *Nature* 524 (2015), 97–101.

Chen, Shu-Jinf Jean 'Fujifilm looks to expand in life sciences with Toyama Chemical', *Forbes Magazine* (February 13, 2018). www.forbes.com/2008/02/13/fujifilm-toyama-update-markets-equity-cx_jc_0213markets04.html#6e91c6bb1529

Davis Nicola 'Antibiotic shortage puts patients at risk, doctors fear', *The Observer* (July 1, 2017). www.theguardian.com/society/2017/jul/01/antibiotic-shortage-puts-patients-at-risk

Desclaux, Alice, and Julienne Anoko 'L'anthropologie engagée dans la lutte contre Ebola (2014–2016): Approches, contributions et nouvelles questions', *Santé publique* 29 (4) (2017), 477–485.

Epelboin, Alain 'L'anthropologie dans la réponse aux épidémies: Science, savoir-faire, ou placébo', *Bulletin de l'AMADES* 78 (2009). http://journals.openedition.org/amades/1060

Eybpoosh, Sana, Ali Akbar Haghdoost, Estphan Mostafavi, et al. 'Molecular epidemiology of infectious diseases', *Electronic Physician* 9 (2017), 5149–5158.

Faria, Nuno R., Andrew Rambaut, Marc A. Suchard, Guy Baele, Trevor Bedford, Melissa J. Ward, Andrew J. Tatem, et al. 'The early spread and epidemic ignition of HIV1 in human populations', *Science* 346 (2014), 56–61.

Frieden, Thomas R., Inger Damon, Beth P. Bell, Thomas Kenyon, and Stuart Nichol 'Ebola 2014 – New challenges, new global response and responsibility', *New England Journal of Medicine* 371 (2014), 1177–1180.

Geissler, Wenzel, and Catherine Molyneux *Evidence, Ethos and Experiment: The Anthropology and History of Medical Research in Africa* (London: Berghahn Books, 2011).

Georges-Courbot, Marie-Claude, Anthony Sanchez, Chang-Yong Lu, Sylvain Baize, Eric Leroy, Joseph Lansout-Soukate, Carole Tévi-Bénissan, et al. 'Isolation and phylogenetic characterization of Ebola viruses causing different outbreaks in Gabon', *Emerging Infectious Diseases* 3 (1) (1997), 59–62.

Gire, Stephen K., Augustine Goba, Kristian G. Andersen, Rachel S. G. Sealfon, Daniel J. Park, Lansana Kanneh, Simbirie Jalloh, et al. 'Genomic surveillance elucidates Ebola virus origin and transmission during the 2014 outbreak', *Science* 345 (2014), 1369–1372.

Goguen, Adam, and Catherine Bolten 'Ebola through a glass, darkly: Ways of knowing the state and each other', *Anthropological Quarterly* 90 (2) (2017), 423–449.

Gomez-Temesio, Veronica, and Frédéric Le Marcis 'La mise en camp de la Guinée: Ébola et experience postcoloniale', *l'Homme* 222 (2017), 57–90.

Hochschild, Adam *King Leopold's Ghost: A Story of Greed, Terror, and Heroism in Colonial Africa* (Boston: Mariner Books, 2006).

Hooper, Edward *The River: A Journey to the Source of HIV and AIDS* (Harmondsworth: Penguin Books, 1999).

Karina, Yusim, M. Peeters, O. G. Pybus, T. Bhattacharya, E. Delaporte, C. Mulanga, M. Muldoon, J. Theiler, and B. Korber 'Using human immunodeficiency virus type 1 sequences to infer historical features of the acquired immune deficiency syndrome epidemic and human immunodeficiency virus evolution', *Philosophical Transactions of the Royal Society of London, Series B* 356 (1410) (2001), 855–866.

Keck, Frédéric, and Christos Lynteris 'Zoonosis: Prospects and challenges for medical anthropology', *Medicine Anthropology Theory* 5 (3) (2018), 1–14.

Kilbourne, Jean-Marc Froment, Magdalena Bermejo, et al. 'Multiple Ebola virus transmission events and rapid decline of central African wildlife', *Science* 303 (2004), 387–390.

Lachenal, Guillaume, Céline Lefève, and Vinh-Kim Nguyen *La Médecine du Tri: Histoire, Éthique, Anthropologie* (Paris: Presses Universitaires de France, 2014).

Landecker, Hannah 'Antibiotic resistance and the biology of history', *Body & Society* 22 (4) (2016), 19–52.

Le Marcis, Frédéric, and Vinh-Kim Nguyen 'Yalta in West Africa: An Ebola photo essay', *Limn* 5 (2015). https://limn.it/articles/an-ebola-photo-essay/

Leach, Melissa 'Ebola in Guinea – people, patterns, and puzzles', *The Lancet Global Health Blog* (2014). http://globalhealth.thelancet.com/2014/04/03/ebola-guinea-people-patterns-and-puzzles

Lena, P. and Luciw P. 'Polio vaccine and retroviruses', *Philosophical Transactions of the Royal Society of London Series B* 356 (1410) (2001), 841–844.

Leroy, Eric M., Pierre Rouquet, Pierre Formenty, Sandrine Souquière, Annelisa Kilbourne, Jean-Marc Froment, Magdalena Bermejo, Sheilag Smit, William Karesh, Robert Swanepoel, Sherif R. Zaki, Pierre E. Rollin 'Multiple Ebola Virus Transmission Events and Rapid Decline of Central African Wildlife', *Science* 303 (16 January 2004) 387–390.

Lock, Margaret, and Vinh-Kim Nguyen *An Anthropology of Biomedicine*, 2nd edition (London: Wiley-Blackwell, 2018).

Lock, Margaret *Twice Dead: Organ Transplants and the Reinvention of Death* (Berkeley, CA: The University of California Press, 2001).

MacPhail, Theresa 'The viral gene: An undead metaphor recoding life', *Science as Culture* 13 (3) (2010), 325–345.

Marx, P. A., P. G. Alcabes, and E. Drucker 'Serial human passage of simian immunodeficiency virus by unsterile injections and the emergence of epidemic human immunodeficiency virus in Africa', *Philosophical Transactions of the Royal Society of London, Series B*, 356 (1410) (2001), 911–920.

Mate, Suzanne E., Jeffrey R. Kugelman, Tolbert G. Nyenswah, Jason T. Ladner, Michael R. Wiley, Thierry Cordier-Lassalle, Athalia Christie, et al. 'Molecular evidence of sexual transmission of Ebola virus', *New England Journal of Medicine* 373 (2015), 2448–2454.

Moran, Mary 'Missing bodies and secret funerals: The production of "safe and dignified burials" in the Liberian Ebola crisis', *Anthropological Quarterly* 90 (2) (2017), 399–421.

Pépin, J., M. Lavoie, O. G. Pybus, R. Pouillot, Y. Foupouapouognigni, D. Rousset, A. C. Labbé, and R. Njouom 'Risk factors for hepatitis C virus transmission in colonial Cameroon', *Clinical Infectious Diseases* 51 (7) (2010), 768–776.

Ragonnet-Cronin, Manon, Jackson Celia, Bradley-Steward Amanda, et al. 'Recent and rapid transmission of HIV among people who inject drugs in Scotland revealed through phylogenetic analysis', *The Journal of Infectious Diseases* 217 (12) (2018), 1875–1882.

Schmitt, Carl *Political Theology: Four Chapters on the Concept of Sovereignty* (Chicago, IL: The University of Chicago Press, 2005 [1934]).

Sharp, Paul M., George M. Shaw, and Beatrice Hahn 'Simian immunodeficiency virus infection of chimpanzees', *Journal of Virology* 79 (2005), 3891–3902.

Shepler, Susan ' "We know who is eating the Ebola money!": Corruption, the state, and the Ebola response', *Anthropological Quarterly* 90 (2) (2017), 451–473.

Stadtfeld Chistrophe, Hollway James, and Block Per 'Dynamic network actor models: Investigating coordination ties through time', *Sociological Methodology* (2017), 1–40.

Strickland, G. Thomas. 'Liver disease in Egypt: Hepatitis C superseded schistosomiasis as a result of iatrogenic and biological factors', *Hepatology* 43 (5) (2006), 915–922.

Wilkinson, Annie 'Emerging disease or emerging diagnosis?: Lassa fever and Ebola in Sierra Leone', *Anthropological Quarterly* 90 (2017), 369–397.

World Health Organization 'Origins of the 2014 Ebola epidemic: One year into the Ebola epidemic' (January 2015). www.who.int/csr/disease/ebola/one-year-report/virus-origin/en/

Yousuke, Furuta, Kazumi Takahashi, Kimiyasu Shiraki, Kenichi Sakamoto, Donald F. Smee, Dale L. Barnard, Brian B. Gowen, Justin G. Julander, and John D. Morrey 'T-705 (favipiravir) and related compounds: Novel broad-spectrum inhibitors of RNA viral infections', *Antiviral Research* 82 (2009), 95–102.

Index